CARDIOVASCULAR
HEALTH

Also in the Your Health Series:

CARDIOVASCULAR HEALTH

LIVING YOUR BEST WITH A HEALTHY HEART

Martin Juneau M.D., M.Ps., FRCP(C)

Foreword by Pierre Lavoie
Translated by Barbara Sandilands

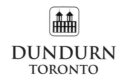

DUNDURN
TORONTO

Printer: Friesens
Cover Image: gettyimages.ca/Alija

Library and Archives Canada Cataloguing in Publication

Juneau, Martin, 1953-
[Coeur pour la vie. English]
Cardiovascular health : living your best with a healthy heart / Martin
Juneau, M.D., M.Ps., FRCP(C) ; foreword by Pierre Lavoie ; translated by
Barbara Sandilands.

Translation of: Un coeur pour la vie.
Includes bibliographical references.
Issued in print and electronic formats.

ISBN 978-1-4597-3893-5 (softcover).--ISBN 978-1-4597-3894-2 (PDF).-- ISBN 978-1-4597-3895-9 (EPUB)

1. Cardiovascular system--Diseases--Prevention. 2. Heart--Diseases--
Prevention. I. Sandilands, Barbara, translator II. Title. III. Title: Coeur
pour la vie. English.

RC672.J8613 2018   616.1'205   C2017-906931-4
                                             C2017-906932-2

1   2   3   4   5   22   21   20   19   18

 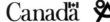 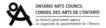

We acknowledge the support of the **Canada Council for the Arts**, which last year invested $153 million to bring the arts to Canadians throughout the country, and the **Ontario Arts Council** for our publishing program. We also acknowledge the financial support of the **Government of Ontario**, through the **Ontario Book Publishing Tax Credit** and the **Ontario Media Development Corporation**, and the **Government of Canada**.

Nous remercions le **Conseil des arts du Canada** de son soutien. L'an dernier, le Conseil a investi 153 millions de dollars pour mettre de l'art dans la vie des Canadiennes et des Canadiens de tout le pays.

Care has been taken to trace the ownership of copyright material used in this book. The author and the publisher welcome any information enabling them to rectify any references or credits in subsequent editions.

— *J. Kirk Howard, President*

The publisher is not responsible for websites or their content unless they are owned by the publisher.

Printed and bound in Canada.

VISIT US AT

 dundurn.com | @dundurnpress | dundurnpress | dundurnpress

Dundurn
3 Church Street, Suite 500
Toronto, Ontario, Canada
M5E 1M2

This book is dedicated to Dr. Paul David, founder of the Montreal Heart Institute, a great humanist and visionary doctor, who firmly believed in prevention and who has inspired my entire career.

This book is also dedicated to all staff at this highly specialized hospital, who have been caring for patients from Quebec and elsewhere for over sixty years, always with unfailing dedication.

Contents

A Trailblazer in a White Coat

I'm extremely proud to write the foreword for this book by Martin Juneau. This is an opportunity for me to pay homage not only to the remarkable work he has been doing for years in the field of medical prevention but also to the exceptional qualities of this man I look on as a friend.

Dr. Martin Juneau is a trailblazer — there's no other word for it. Thirty years ago, he chose to focus his energies on preventive medicine. It wasn't easy, at a time when the whole system revolved around curative medicine, to convince patients to change behaviours harmful to their health.

You need strong convictions, unwavering perseverance, and enormous credibility. You need someone like Martin Juneau, who has succeeded over the years in sowing in people's minds the seeds of the idea that our lifestyle habits have a direct effect on our current and future quality of life. I'm delighted to be following his example.

As far as I know, Martin was the first person to sound the alarm in the media about obesity, high blood pressure, and everything else that can negatively affect cardiovascular health. At the time, I watched him from afar, never suspecting that one day I would have the privilege of working with him.

We first met in the fall of 1998. Germain Thibault, my current associate, who was then a producer at Radio-Canada, had contacted me to invite me to participate in a news story on the Ironman competition. He wanted to have my cardiorespiratory condition assessed by an authority — cardiologist Martin Juneau.

That was the beginning of a long collaboration. When we set up the board of directors for the Grand défi Pierre Lavoie — the Pierre Lavoie Challenge — Martin was the first to agree to be a part of this new adventure, demonstrating that the trailblazer in his soul is always ready to lend a hand for a cause he believes in.

Today, when I have questions about the results of a new medical study, need statistics, or have to validate information for my lectures, I call Martin. He's my scientific reference, and I think that

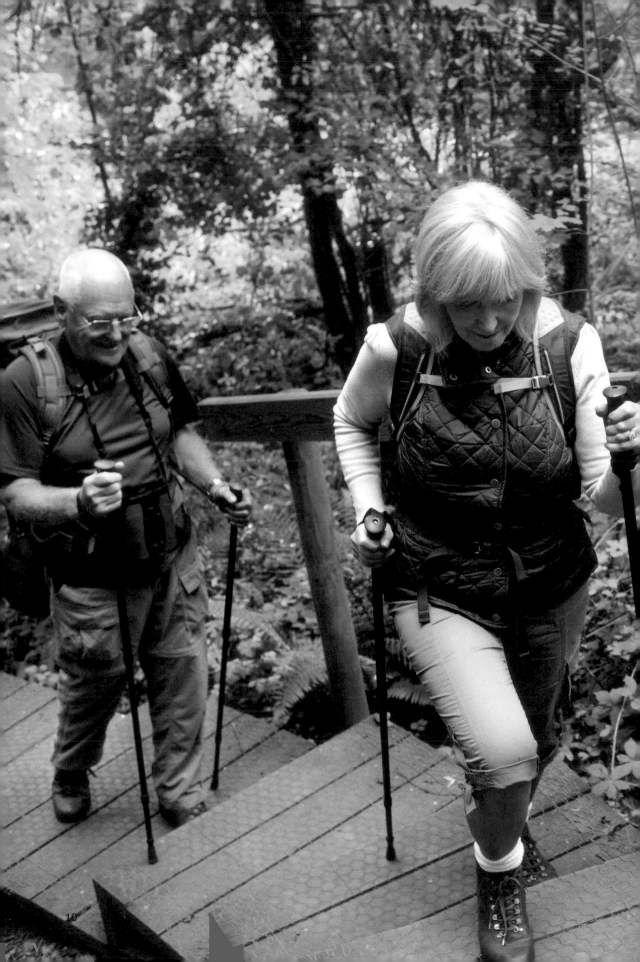

Cardiovascular Health is going to make him one for many people.

In his book, Martin presents the most recent research on the prevention of chronic diseases in a way that everyone can understand. Science applied to good old common sense is what gives *Cardiovascular Health* so much vital energy. After reading it, you'll know exactly what you have to do to maintain a high quality of life based on a few basic principles.

I'm glad we now have a book dealing with preventive medicine in a way that makes us realize that prevention is easier than we think. Interviews and video clips are all very well, but a book can go much further to raise awareness — especially a book like this one, written by Quebec's prevention pioneer. I'm convinced that if you put the advice you find here into practice, you'll feel better, and so will our society, for life!

Pierre Lavoie
Ironman and Co-Founder
of the Pierre Lavoie Challenge

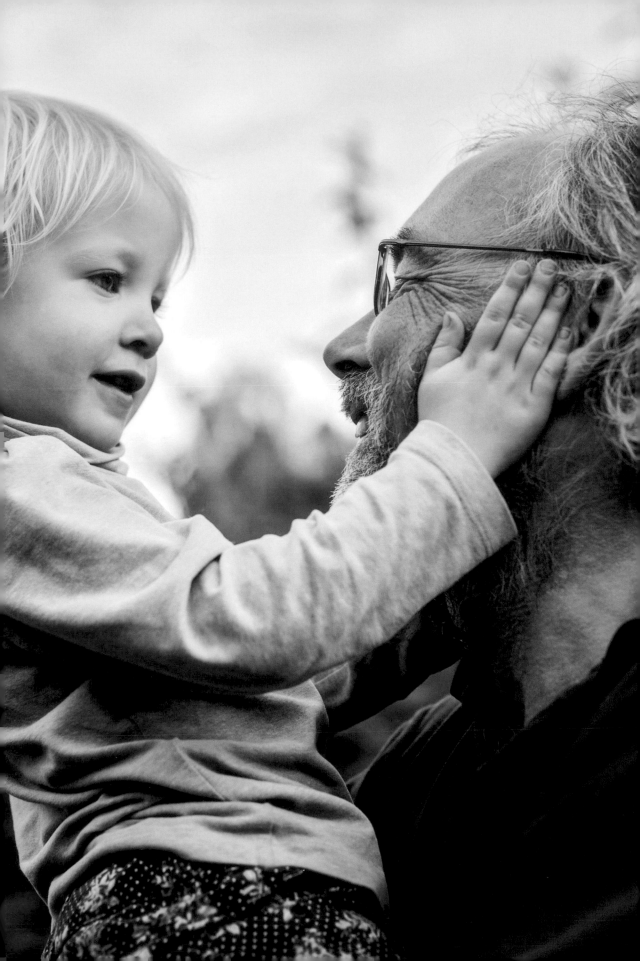

Chronic Disease Prevention for a Better, Longer Life

Although we all agree that an ounce of prevention is worth a pound of cure, in everyday life we place our hopes much more on curing diseases than on preventing them. Governments can be defeated because of problems related to the healthcare system, like waiting lists that are too long or overflowing emergency rooms, but never because there isn't enough prevention.

It's therefore not accidental that our healthcare system is mainly oriented toward treating diseases while prevention is overlooked. According to the Canadian Institute for Health Information, in 2013 only 5.1% of the total healthcare expenditure in Canada was for public health, which encompasses activities related to health promotion and prevention, a proportion clearly inadequate to counter the damage caused by smoking, obesity, and a sedentary lifestyle.

Like most of my colleagues, I chose to specialize in cardiology because I wanted to save lives and alleviate the symptoms of patients who have cardiovascular disease.

Medical progress achieved during the past century has given modern medicine an impressive arsenal of drugs, imaging techniques, and intervention procedures that have prevented an incalculable number of premature deaths and contributed to an increased life expectancy.

Although this progress is impressive, cardiologists are the first to realize the limits of this curative approach every day. For example, even though we can usually save patients in the acute phase of a heart attack, it's much more difficult to treat the underlying causes of the attack — the process of atherosclerosis that attacks the interior of the coronary arteries, which nourish the cardiac muscle. As a result, even if they are out of danger in the short term, patients who have had an acute heart attack and do not deal with the problems that caused the disease (poor diet, sedentariness, smoking) risk having a second heart attack and, ultimately, developing heart failure, which will undermine their quality of life.

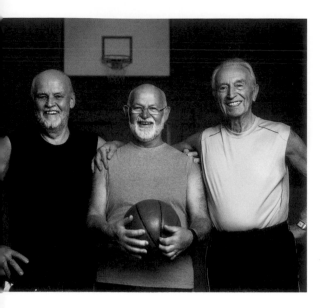

In other words, modern medicine is excellent and unequalled for treating events that suddenly put a person's life in danger, but its effectiveness remains limited in the face of chronic diseases that develop insidiously over decades.

Experts agree that lifestyle is one of the main factors in the development of chronic diseases. For example, the decrease in mortality observed since the 1970s in people with cardiovascular disease is due not only to medical advances but also to improvement in certain lifestyle habits, in particular the significant decline in smoking in the last fifty years. Unfortunately, it's thought that these recent gains will be cancelled out by the negative effects of obesity and junk food, and we are already beginning to glimpse the first signs of an increase in the incidence of cardiovascular disease in young people. In an editorial that appeared recently in the medical journal *JAMA Cardiology*, Dr. Donald M. Lloyd-Jones of the Department of Preventive Medicine at Northwestern University

in Chicago underlined that the gains made in the last fifty years will be erased by the largest epidemic of chronic diseases in the history of humanity. Since 1985 we have, in fact, witnessed steady increases in obesity and diabetes, affecting every age group in society and contributing to a resurgence in cardiovascular disease, especially in young adults. What's more, recent data show that the incidence of heart attacks has not decreased in the last ten years in men ages 30 to 54 and that it has actually increased among women in this age group.

This is an alarming situation. One serious problem our society faces is that healthy life expectancy, without incapacitating illness, has not increased as fast as total life expectancy. For example, in Canada life expectancy is 79 years of age for men and 83 for women, whereas healthy life expectancy is just 69 for men and 71 for women — a difference of ten and twelve years, respectively. A great many people will spend the last ten or twelve years of their lives in poor health despite medical progress. This situation may get worse in coming years because of the dramatic increase in obesity and the chronic diseases resulting from it.

Fortunately, despite the seriousness of the problem, many studies have shown that the majority of chronic diseases, and especially cardiovascular disease, can be avoided or greatly delayed by making simple lifestyle changes. These studies tell us that we must not just give up: we can avoid the premature onset of diseases associated with aging and thus dramatically improve our quality of life. Our lifespan has its limits, but taking action to shorten the period of late-life disability as much as possible lets us maximize the potential of human life.

For more than three decades of clinical practice and research at the Montreal Heart Institute (MHI) and its prevention centre (the EPIC Centre), I have been in a position to see, every day, the degree to which people who decide to profoundly change their lifestyle can improve their health and quality of life. The effects are often impressive: many patients who complete a secondary prevention program after a heart attack or surgery say they are in much better shape than before their cardiac event because it triggered major changes in their lifestyle.

The aim of this book is to share with you my belief that chronic diseases, and cardiovascular disease in particular, are not inevitable and that it's possible, by changing our habits, to live a long and healthy life.

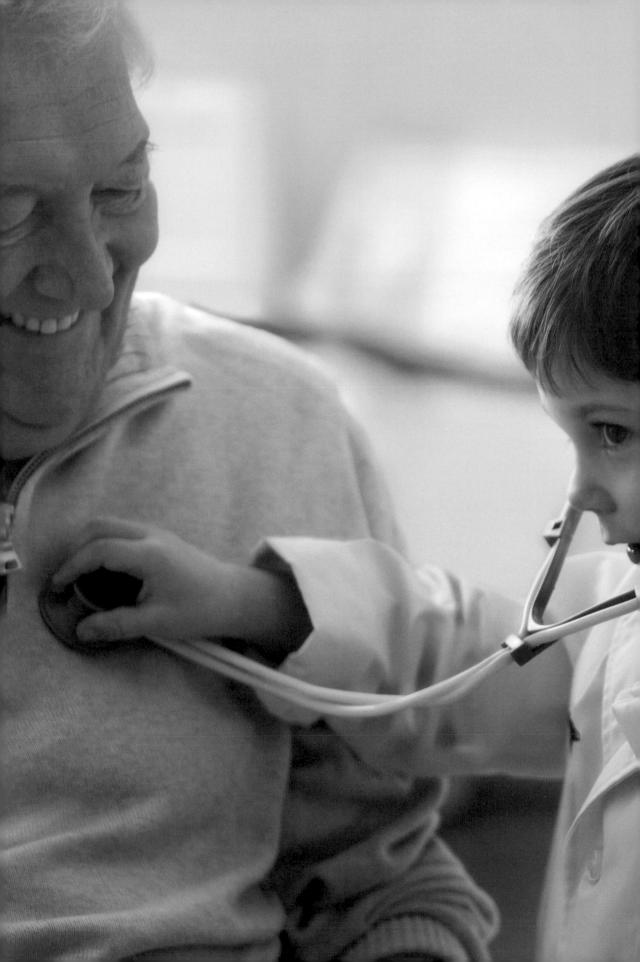

CHAPTER 1

Healthy Life Expectancy and Chronic Diseases

In Canada, as in all industrialized countries, the life expectancy of a child born today is about eighty years, or almost twice what it was 150 years ago (Figure 1).

The first factor that explains this phenomenal increase in longevity is the notable decline in premature mortality during childhood and young adulthood. This success is due in large part to improvements in health conditions, as well as to the discovery of antibiotics and vaccines; these discoveries led to the eradication of many kinds of bacteria and viruses that caused infections and serious illnesses, thus saving innumerable lives.

However, this increase in longevity would not have reached current levels without a decrease in mortality at more advanced ages brought about by enormous medical advances in treating many diseases. Surgical procedures (which are increasingly sophisticated), organ transplants, drug therapies, and early diagnosis using imaging, to name just a few — all these advances enable us to save a large number of people from premature death and thus add many years to their lives.

Dramatic though it is, this increase in life expectancy nonetheless hides a more sombre reality: we may live longer, but the extra years are very often characterized by illness and suffering. For example, men born in Canada in 1990 will live to age 73 on average, but their state of health will begin to deteriorate eight years earlier, at age 65.

For those born in 2013, the average age at death climbs to 79, with health problems making their appearance ten years earlier, at 69. In other words, even though life expectancy has increased by six years in the last twenty-five years, the years in good health have not increased at the same rate, meaning that Canadian men will have

INCREASE IN LIFE EXPECTANCY DURING THE NINETEENTH AND TWENTIETH CENTURIES

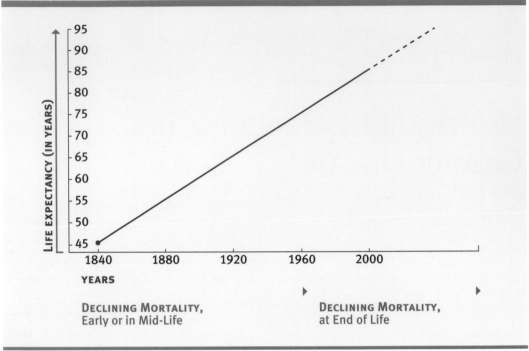

FIGURE 1

Adapted from Oeppen, 2002, and Kirkwood, 2008

to live, on average, one more year in poor health. And this is not an isolated case: according to World Health Organization (WHO) statistics, healthy life expectancy for most people on the planet is, on average, ten years less than their total life expectancy. Obviously, this discrepancy means that increased life expectancy will offer substantially fewer benefits: the main goal is not to live longer at any cost but rather to enjoy those extra years and make the most of our brief existence.

Are years of life in poor health inevitable, a kind of ransom to pay for the phenomenal increase in longevity over the past century? Pessimists will say yes, and that it's better to die younger than to spend the last ten to fifteen years of our lives growing

old in misery, faced with a mediocre quality of life that leaves us unable to live normally, while often imposing a burden on those close to us. I do not share this fatalistic view, since many studies on aging show that it's possible to prolong not only total life expectancy but, more importantly, *healthy* life expectancy.

Researcher James F. Fries, at Stanford University, has documented this very well in his research: he observed a reduction of seven to twelve years in the period of late-life disability among people who engaged in moderate physical activity. Similarly, a major study begun in 1986 among former University of Pennsylvania students showed that participants who performed moderate physical activity, did not smoke,

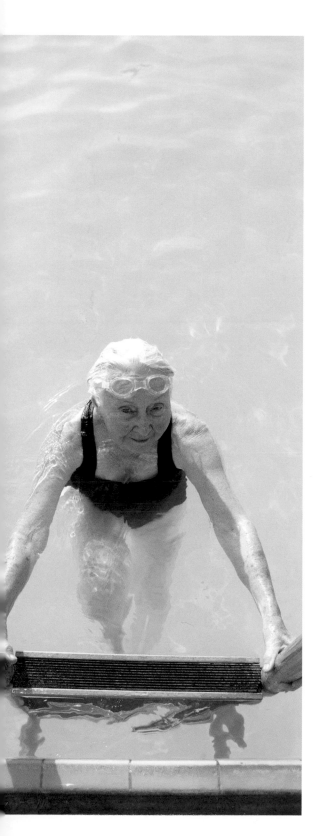

and maintained a healthy weight delayed late-life disability by more than seven years. Many similar studies have since been published.

PERCEIVED DECLINE IN LIFE EXPECTANCY IN YOUNGER GENERATIONS

While baby boomers have a healthy life expectancy shorter than their total life expectancy, young people are facing another reality: lower life expectancy as a result of the consequences of the obesity epidemic. Researcher S. Jay Olshansky and his colleagues predicted ten years ago that young Americans born in the 1990s might be the first generation in a century to experience a decrease in life expectancy: they might actually not live as long as their parents. Indeed, the significant gains made in the last fifty years could be wiped out by the consequences of obesity. Whereas between 1961 and 1983 life expectancy increased steadily in all American states, between 1983 and 1999, life expectancy for men living in those states most affected by obesity *decreased.* This decrease in longevity is almost certainly going to accelerate in today's younger generations, since rates of obesity have continued to rise in recent years in the United States and Canada. As David Ludwig, a pediatrician and endocrinologist at Harvard University, has said, medical advances are relatively effective in preventing premature death from obesity that develops at about 45 years of age, diabetes at about 55, and cardiovascular disease at about 65. It will be more and more difficult and expensive, however, to treat the harmful consequences of obesity,

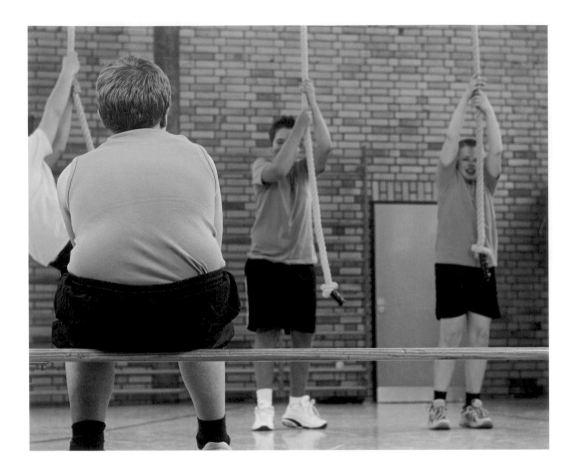

because this sequence of events is now beginning in childhood and adolescence. It's therefore crucial to attack this societal problem quickly through a comprehensive, not just medical, approach. Measures must be taken by all sectors of society to change environments that are toxic to health.

CHRONIC DISEASES

In September 2011, the United Nations (UN) held a summit on the prevention of chronic diseases, also known as "non-communicable diseases." This was a rare event, only the second time in the UN's entire history that a meeting of this size was called on a health issue (the first concerned AIDS and took place in 2000), clearly reflecting the huge challenge posed by these diseases. Contrary to what most people think, a sizable proportion of the mortality attributed to chronic diseases is *premature*; in other words, these diseases do not just affect very old people but also people in the prime of life, with major social and economic consequences. Taken together, diseases of the cardiovascular or respiratory systems, type 2 diabetes, cancer, and neurodegenerative diseases (Alzheimer's and other dementias) are responsible for the majority of deaths worldwide, both in wealthy countries and in countries in economic transition.

As a result of the globalization of trade and the spread of the Western way of life, chronic diseases have replaced malnutrition as the main cause of premature death and disability in developing countries. In China, for example, 90% of deaths are caused by chronic diseases, which especially affect people from 30 to 59 years of age. Note that three hundred million people smoke and 160 million people have high blood pressure in China, two major causes of cardiovascular disease and cancer. The future looks bleak in a country where 20% of children and adolescents are obese as a direct consequence of adopting a Western lifestyle, especially in China's big cities; currently, rural areas remain largely free from chronic diseases. Dr. Barry Popkin, an economics professor at the University of North Carolina and a specialist in health economics issues in developing countries, predicts that the poor diet and sedentary lifestyle that have taken hold in China and are spreading very quickly will overwhelm the Chinese health system and slow economic growth. He believes that the costs associated with chronic diseases will represent between 4% and 8% of the country's entire economy. To this must be added the enormous costs related to the harmful effects of air pollution on the health of the Chinese.

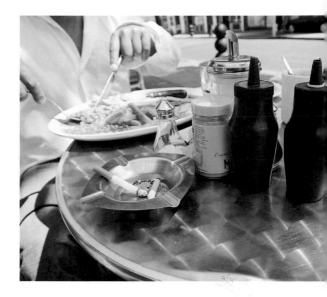

According to the director-general of the WHO, Dr. Margaret Chan, chronic diseases are a human and economic catastrophe that risks greatly endangering the development of every nation, even the wealthiest. Just like climate change, chronic diseases are one of the biggest challenges of the twenty-first century.

Since chronic diseases, and especially cardiovascular disease, can be treated, all health expenditures are aimed at *treatments*, while the root *causes*, related mainly to lifestyle, are not taken into account. According to the WHO, as many as 80% of cases of heart disease, stroke, and type 2 diabetes, and as many as 30% of cancers could be avoided by eliminating risk factors shared by these diseases — smoking, poor diet, and sedentariness.

The scope of this challenge is especially obvious in Canada, where chronic diseases alone, mainly cardiovascular disease, cancer, and respiratory diseases, are responsible for roughly 75% of all deaths annually (Figure 2).

Not only are these diseases a human tragedy, they also all place enormous pressures on our health care systems. In Canada, cardiovascular diseases are the primary cause of hospitalizations and surgical operations, as well as being the category of diseases whose direct costs are highest. According to a report by the CIRANO group, the proportion of Quebec's budget dedicated to health care now makes up 49% of all government expenditures. If growth in healthcare expenditures continues at the same rate, about 2% per year

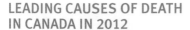

LEADING CAUSES OF DEATH IN CANADA IN 2012

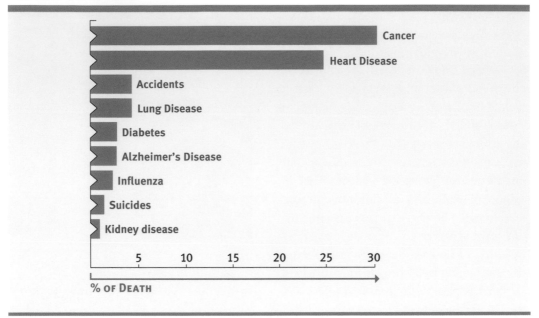

FIGURE 2   Source: Statistics Canada

(an optimistic estimate), the share of the provincial budget dedicated to the healthcare system will reach 70% by 2030 (a similar study, authored by leading economists, projected healthcare spending in Ontario will account for 80 percent of total program spending by 2030). This is, of course, an unsustainable situation that will endanger a number of the government's essential mandates, such as education, other social measures, and infrastructure.

The fight against chronic diseases is complicated by the fact that these diseases develop very slowly, often without obvious symptoms, and that the people affected are completely ignorant of the factors responsible for their development. The violent nature of a heart attack or stroke can lead us to believe that these diseases occur

suddenly, but they are merely the conclusion of a very long process, during which atheromatous plaques develop gradually on the walls of blood vessels. Inflammation developing on these atheromatous plaques can cause the plaque to rupture and may lead to the formation of a clot. If the clot is big enough, it can completely block the artery and cause an obstruction that results in a heart attack that can be fatal. Modern medical feats, like rapid dilation of the blockage, often succeed in saving the patient's life; this may give the impression he or she has been "cured," but unfortunately this is not the case. A heart attack is just the visible sign of a much bigger problem that the patient must deal with; otherwise, the risk of recurrence will be high. To conquer chronic diseases, especially cardiovascular diseases, we must first prevent their development.

The means exist to do this, and they are not at all extreme or inaccessible. A great many studies have clearly proven that just five simple lifestyle changes can significantly reduce cardiovascular disease (Figure 3).

The effectiveness of these behavioural changes in preventing heart attacks is striking: while some of the most commonly prescribed drugs for preventing cardiovascular disease (see Chapter 9) only reduce the absolute risk of a coronary event in *primary* prevention by 1%, the combination of these five factors, on the other hand, results in a quite remarkable 85% decrease in absolute risk (Figure 4).

Similar results have been observed in women. Worldwide, a simple change in habits to include these five behaviours could result in a gain of fourteen years of life.

Although they are within everyone's reach, these lifestyle changes are ignored by the majority of the population in industrialized countries. For example, 60% of Canadians do not consume at least five servings of fruit and vegetables a day, 85% do not get at least 2.5 hours of moderately intense physical activity a week, 66% are overweight (including 25% who are obese), and almost 20% still smoke. That leaves only 3% of the population that has adopted these five behaviours!

Yet many major studies have proven the remarkable effectiveness of better lifestyle habits. For example, a Dutch study of thirty-three thousand men and women in good health ages 20 to 70 showed that people who combined the five positive behaviours in Figure 3 decreased by 85%

LIFESTYLE FACTORS ASSOCIATED WITH A REDUCTION IN RISK OF HEART ATTACK IN MEN

Preventive Factors

1. Eat a healthy diet (more plants and whole grains, fewer added sugars, fewer processed foods, less processed meat and red meat).

2. Maintain a normal body weight (waist circumference: <100 cm for men and <88 cm for women).

3. Don't smoke.

4. Get regular physical activity (30 minutes per day of walking or cycling, for example).

5. Drink alcohol in moderation (from 10 to 30 g — one or two drinks — per day).

FIGURE 3   Source: Adapted from Åkesson, 2014

their risk of having a *premature* stroke, as well as considerably increasing their *healthy* life expectancy. Adopting a healthier lifestyle is thus a very effective way not only to prolong our life expectancy but especially — and this is the most important thing — to prolong our *healthy* life expectancy.

COLLATERAL EFFECTS

The changes in lifestyle described in this book do not prevent just cardiovascular diseases. For about ten years now, I have noticed that my patients are much less

DECLINE IN INCIDENCE OF HEART ATTACK IN MEN WITH ONE OR MORE LIFESTYLE-RELATED PROTECTIVE FACTORS

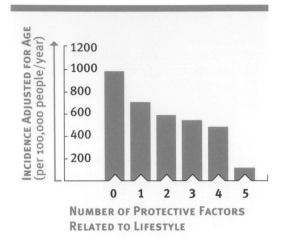

FIGURE 4   Source: Adapted from Åkesson, 2014

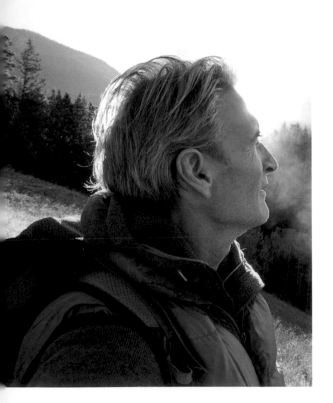

afraid of dying of a heart attack than from cancer or Alzheimer's disease. They have the impression that a heart attack is a "good death," quite quick and relatively painless, whereas they are terrified of the idea of losing their intellectual faculties and ending their life in a nursing home, entirely dependent on others.

But studies done in recent years have clearly shown that the lifestyle habits associated with a reduction in risk for cardiovascular diseases also have a preventive effect against many cancers (especially colon, lung, breast, and prostate cancers), as well as against neurodegenerative diseases, like Alzheimer's disease. Furthermore, we now know that a large proportion of dementias are directly linked to our cardiovascular health and that we can, as a result, prevent their onset simply by adopting lifestyle habits known to decrease the incidence of cardiovascular disease.

WHAT ABOUT GENETICS?

We often try to associate a long life expectancy with some kind of "longevity gene" that might protect some people from the disease. Yet many studies have clearly shown that the "secret" of people who live long lives is not genetic; for example, a recent study could not find any notable difference in the gene sequence of supercentenarian people that could explain their incredible longevity (110 years and more). Except in the case of some rare genetic diseases, fate is not determined at birth: research in the last fifty years in the fields of nutrition and physical activity shows that our diet and our daily activities strongly influence our health and can more than compensate for poor genetics.

Indeed, the science of epigenetics, the ways our genes express themselves, confirms that lifestyle habits have an effect on "undesirable" and "desirable" genes. In other words, if your parents suffered from a severe cardiovascular disease, you are not condemned to endure the same fate, since your lifestyle habits can modify the activation of your "bad" genes. In short, good lifestyle habits activate the "good" genes and deactivate the "bad."

TELOMERES AND LIFESTYLE HABITS

Our genes are DNA sequences dispersed along twenty-three pairs of chromosomes located inside the nuclei of our cells. These chromosomes have "caps" at each end called telomeres, which protect the genetic material from damage during cell division (Figure 5).

As we age, our telomeres gradually shorten, so their length is an indicator of how much longer we have to live and of our overall health. The longer they are, the more healthy years we have left; the shorter they are, the closer we are to death and the more we have various forms of disability. Dr. Elizabeth Blackburn received the Nobel Prize in Physiology or Medicine in 2009 for her work on telomeres. In collaboration with Dr. Blackburn, Dr. Dean Ornish showed that a lifestyle behaviour change program followed over five years by an experimental group resulted in participants having longer telomeres, while the telomeres in the control group got shorter (Figure 6). That simple changes in lifestyle habits have such an impact on our DNA integrity shows just how predominant a role our way of life plays in maintaining good health; this is especially true where cardiovascular health is concerned.

TELOMERES

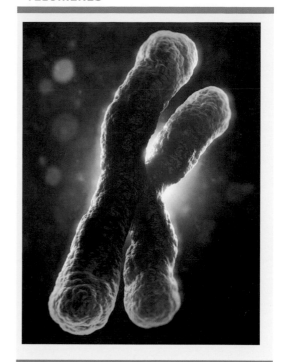

FIGURE 5

IMPACT OF LIFESTYLE ON TELOMERE LENGTH

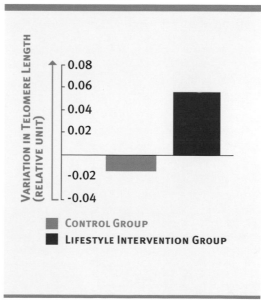

FIGURE 6   Adapted from Ornish et al., 2013

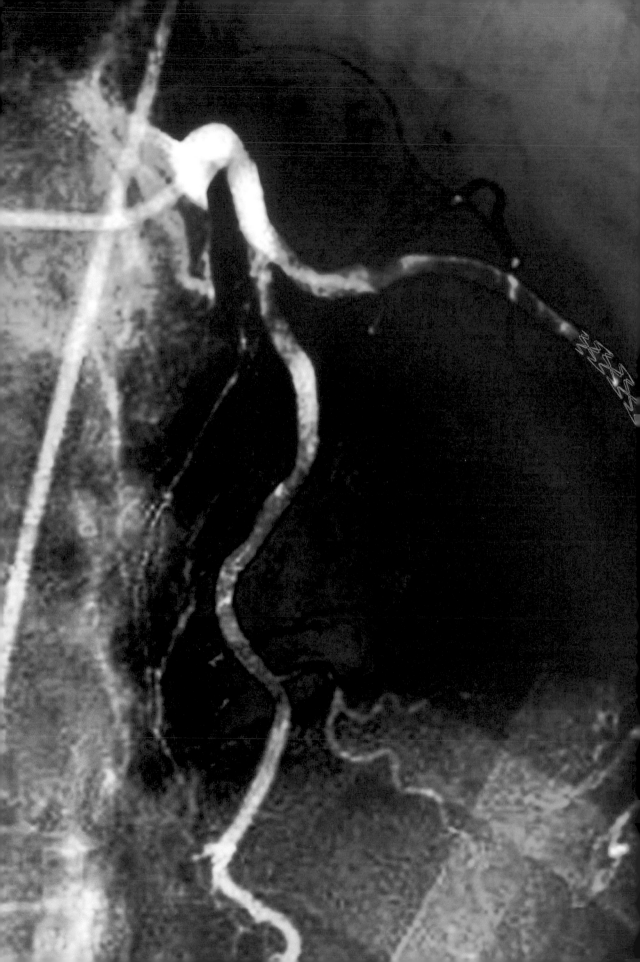

CHAPTER 2

Coronary Disease and Its Treatments

The heart is a hollow muscle the size of your clenched fist whose function is to ensure the constant circulation of blood throughout the entire organism. It's nothing more than a pump that receives venous blood from the vena cava (the right side of the heart) and sends it back through the organism via the aorta (left side) after it has been oxygenated by the lungs (Figure 7).

The heart muscle, or myocardium, receives oxygen through its network of arteries, called coronary arteries, since they form a crown (from the Latin *corona*) around the heart. These arteries are three millimetres in diameter at their root, or roughly the size of a wooden match. Their diameter narrows as the arteries branch out and penetrate the cardiac muscle to provide the oxygen it needs to sustain the constant contraction of the heart (one hundred thousand beats a day, on average). There are two coronary arteries, left and right. The left artery divides rapidly into two main branches: the anterior descending artery irrigates the front of the heart, and the circumflex artery irrigates the left side of the heart (Figure 8). In practice, these two divisions of the left coronary artery are often considered to be two distinct arteries. We often speak of "three-vessel" coronary disease when the right coronary, the left anterior descending, and the circumflex artery are affected. Depending on the number of coronary arteries affected, we refer to one-, two-, or three-vessel heart disease.

This is a simplification just to indicate the extent of the coronary disease; in fact, all the coronary arteries are affected to varying degrees even when only one of them shows a visible blockage.

BLOOD CIRCULATION

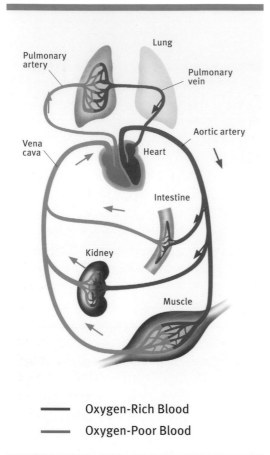

Pulmonary artery

Lung

Pulmonary vein

Aortic artery

Vena cava

Heart

Intestine

Kidney

Muscle

—— Oxygen-Rich Blood
—— Oxygen-Poor Blood

FIGURE 7

CIRCULATORY TRAFFIC JAMS

Coronary disease is very dangerous: when a coronary artery is partially or completely blocked, the myocardial region irrigated by this coronary artery lacks blood and therefore lacks oxygen, a condition known in medical language as *myocardial ischemia* (from the Greek *iskhô*, meaning "to stop," and *haîma*, meaning "blood"). Oxygen is stored inside the hemoglobin in red blood cells. When ischemia lasts too long, about twenty minutes, the cells in the cardiac

muscle begin to die and its functioning is compromised.

Plaques formed by the process of atherosclerosis are what cause coronary blockage (see Chapter 3). In clinical practice, we can see these plaques using an imaging technique called *coronary angiography* (Figure 9). Coronary angiography involves inserting a catheter (a small hollow tube) into the coronary arteries, usually through the radial artery in the wrist, and injecting a radio-opaque solution (so that the interior of the artery can be seen by X-rays) to show where any blockages are located.

These blockages are often located in the forks (where blood circulation is more turbulent), but they can occur anywhere. The more proximal the artery blockage (at the beginning of the artery), the greater the damage will be. As a simple analogy, it's a little like cutting into a tree: if you cut close to the roots, the whole tree will fall; if you cut only near the top, you lose very few branches.

Until the 1990s, it was believed that a heart attack — the total blockage of the coronary artery causing the death of the myocardium irrigated by this artery — was the result of a gradual shrinking of the vessel, caused by steadily growing plaque. It was later noticed, however, that this blockage could be caused suddenly by plaques that were very undeveloped and inconspicuous in angiography exams. These plaques can become inflamed and break apart or erode quickly, leading to the formation of a clot that can partially or totally obstruct blood flow in the artery. This is why you can feel very well one minute and then suddenly be struck down by a heart attack. In summary, when an atherosclerotic plaque ruptures or erodes, a clot forms, the coronary artery becomes completely blocked, and the result is a sudden heart attack.

ARTERIES OF THE HEART

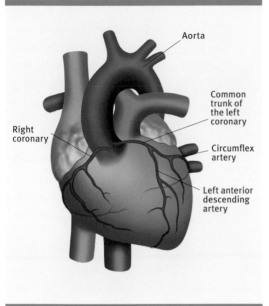

FIGURE 8

BLOCKAGE (STENOSIS) VISUALIZED WITH CORONARY ANGIOGRAPHY

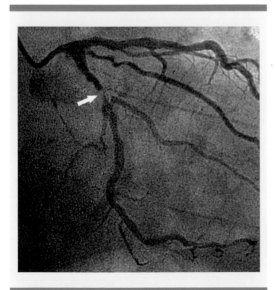

FIGURE 9

WHAT IS ANGINA?

Angina is a pain in the chest, usually in the centre, caused by the narrowing of one or several coronary arteries. This partial blockage (of 60% to 70% of the artery's internal diameter) slows down blood flow, depriving the myocardium of oxygen. Angina usually occurs during exertion (when the heart muscle is working harder and needs more oxygen) and is relieved by rest. For example, someone shovelling snow a little too fast feels pain in the middle of the chest. He stops shovelling, and the pain goes away in a few minutes. If he starts shovelling again, the pain comes back very quickly, in exactly the same place. This pain (very worrisome for the person feeling it) is really a defence mechanism in the body warning us to immediately stop exertion, which is dangerous for the heart muscle. Angina pain may be located only in the middle of the chest, or it may also radiate outward to the left arm, the left shoulder, and sometimes the right shoulder and fists, as well as to the neck and sometimes the jaw (Figure 10). Pain in one of these areas that occurs during exertion and disappears during rest can be a sign of coronary disease. People should consult a doctor as soon as possible when they have this type of discomfort.

Angina pain is often more severe after a meal. Our research team at the Montreal Heart Institute's EPIC Centre has shown that angina pain occurs after minor exertion thirty minutes after a one-thousand-calorie meal. In patients with coronary disease who have stable angina, it's therefore preferable to wait at least ninety minutes before exercising. Similarly, when it's cold outside, and especially when it's windy, our team has observed that exercise done at –8°C and at –20°C is associated with increased angina during exertion.

ANGINA PAIN

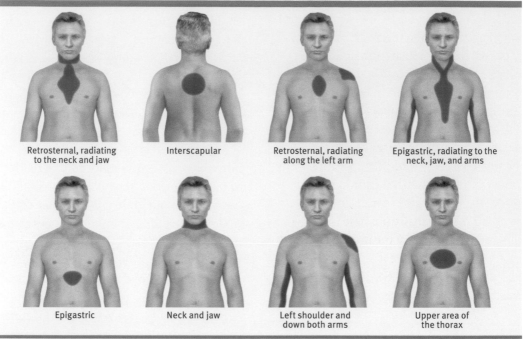

| Retrosternal, radiating to the neck and jaw | Interscapular | Retrosternal, radiating along the left arm | Epigastric, radiating to the neck, jaw, and arms |

| Epigastric | Neck and jaw | Left shoulder and down both arms | Upper area of the thorax |

FIGURE 10

A Heart Attack That Feels Like Indigestion

A few years ago one of my patients called my receptonist to ask for her advice, as he was feeling slight nausea and discomfort in "the pit of the stomach," like "indigestion."

My receptionist, who suspected a heart attack, recommended he call 911, but he preferred to go see his family doctor, who was always available in case of emergency. When the man arrived at the doctor's office, the doctor immediately thought it might indeed be a heart attack; during the examination, the patient went into cardiac arrest. The doctor performed cardiopulmonary resuscitation (CPR) and used a defibrillator to restart the heartbeat. The paramedics arrived very quickly and transported the man to hospital, where an angioplasty was done to unblock the right coronary artery, obstructed by a clot. The patient recovered with no after effects and is still working out at the EPIC Centre.

This true story ended well, but the ending would have been much less happy had each intervenor (the patient, receptionist, and doctor) not thought and acted appropriately.

WHAT'S THE DIFFERENCE BETWEEN ANGINA AND A HEART ATTACK?

Angina occurs when the artery is not totally blocked. During a heart attack the artery is blocked completely and suddenly, accompanied by an immediate lack of blood in an entire part of the myocardium, causing the cells there to die. Most of the time, heart attack pain is very intense. The patient sweats profusely and may even have the impression that death is imminent. This is one of the worst pains seen in medical practice. Often, it's actually possible to diagnose a heart attack just by noting the patient's expression, even before it's confirmed by an electrocardiogram (ECG). The pain, as with angina, is usually in the middle of the chest and may radiate outward to the same areas. In some cases, the heart attack may not be accompanied by pain, especially in very elderly people and people with diabetes. In these cases, it may, for example, resemble nausea, combined with extreme weakness.

HEART ATTACK AND SUDDEN DEATH

We often hear about sudden death, which usually occurs in the first few minutes of the attack as a consequence of a very serious arrhythmia called *ventricular tachycardia* or, most often, because of ventricular fibrillation (Figure 11). The patient discussed earlier experienced this. Sudden death may also occur without a simultaneous heart attack: in this case, ventricular tachycardia that turns into ventricular fibrillation occurs at the site of a scar from an earlier heart attack. This old scar thus causes a kind of short circuit in the heart muscle.

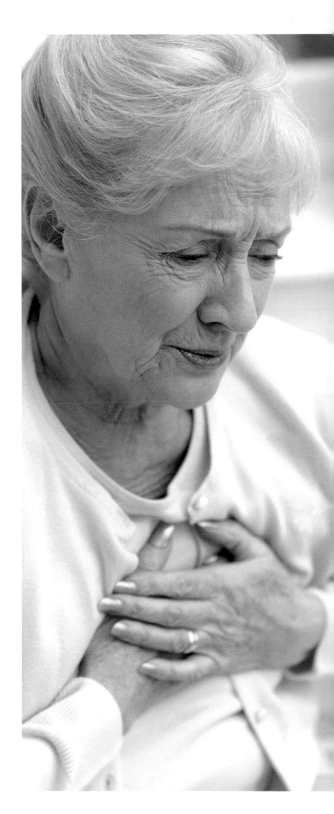

VENTRICULAR FIBRILLATION

During a normal heartbeat, an electric signal goes from the upper chambers (the atria) to the lower chambers (the ventricles), causing the ventricles to contract and blood to circulate. During ventricular fibrillation, there are rapid and irregular electric pulsations in the ventricles; these then contract in a disorderly and inefficient way instead of moving blood through the body.

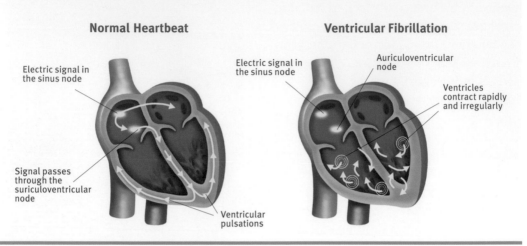

FIGURE 11

Unfortunately, sudden death is often the first sign of coronary disease. This is why it's essential to prevent the onset of coronary disease, since once it has taken hold, if nothing is done to stop it from developing, death can occur unexpectedly.

RESTORING CIRCULATION

You must consult your family doctor right away if you feel discomfort in the chest during physical exertion. The doctor will usually send you to a cardiologist to confirm and clarify the angina diagnosis and begin treatment.

The cardiologist will often have patients do a stress test on a treadmill with an ECG. Usually, after simply asking the patient

questions, the cardiologist already knows it's angina. So why the treadmill? Because the stress test will determine the severity of the angina and its prognosis — its seriousness — as well as whether the patient has to be aggressively or conservatively treated. For example, if the patient finishes the test in seven to ten minutes, depending on the protocol used, and the angina only occurs at a high exertion level, a decision may be made to treat the patient conservatively, with medications rather than angioplasty or an operation.

In this case, it's not a question of eliminating the blockage but of reducing the repercussions of the coronary artery blockage on the myocardium. In other words, the myocardium continues to lack blood during exertion if the patient

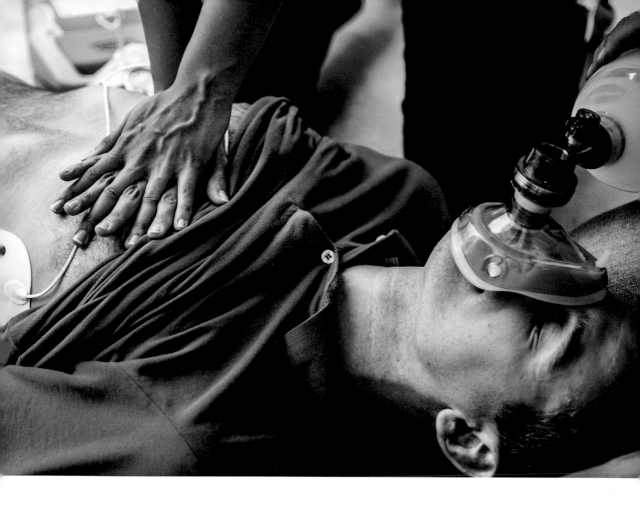

exceeds a certain level, but ischemia (the lack of blood) is reduced because the medication decreases the heart's oxygen consumption or helps increase blood flow to the myocardium. Beta-blockers, for example, reduce the contraction strength of the heart muscle, which means that, during exertion, ischemia and pain are reduced. Calcium antagonists, on the other hand, dilate the coronary arteries. Nitroglycerin, the famous "nitro" that everyone has heard of, causes intense vasodilation of the coronary arteries that relieves pain almost instantly. These drugs are very effective in most cases, and it's common for patients to take an anti-angina drug for years (and sometimes for their life) without having to undergo an intervention like angioplasty or bypass surgery.

On the other hand, if the pain occurs very early in a treadmill stress test and the ECG indicates a significant blockage, the cardiologist may instead decide to examine the coronary arteries directly using angiography (Figure 12).

If the cardiologist was correct, a major blockage will be found during this exam. If so, then the cardiologist may, during the same procedure, insert a thin guidewire as far as the blockage, and then thread onto this guidewire a catheter with a small balloon to dilate the artery. In most cases, the cardiologist will install a tube (also commonly known as a *stent*) to prevent the artery from becoming blocked again. This procedure is done under local anaesthetic (the patient is awake) and takes from forty-five minutes to an hour (Figure 13).

DETECTION OF ANGINA USING A STRESS ECG

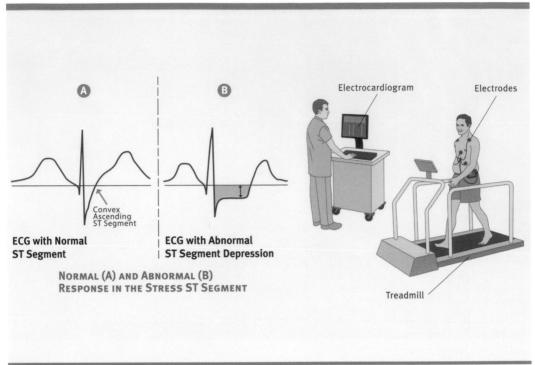

NORMAL (A) AND ABNORMAL (B)
RESPONSE IN THE STRESS ST SEGMENT

ECG with Normal
ST Segment

Convex
Ascending
ST Segment

ECG with Abnormal
ST Segment Depression

Electrocardiogram

Electrodes

Treadmill

FIGURE 12

If the three coronary arteries are severely blocked, the cardiologist may decide, instead of dilating each blockage, to recommend coronary artery bypasses. In this operation, the thorax is opened (the sternum is cut with a special saw). The mammary artery, which supplies the breast with blood, and veins taken from the leg (saphenous veins) are used to create "bridges" over the blockages — hence the name *bypasses* (Figure 14). The mammary artery is attached with stitches to the other side of the blockage in the coronary artery. The saphenous veins are placed between the aorta and the other side of the coronary artery blockage. Each case is different and the cardiologist may decide to dilate three or four blockages rather than having the patient undergo surgery.

There is clearly a huge difference between balloon angioplasty and bypass surgery. Angioplasty is done while the patient is awake and therefore without anaesthesia. The person is conscious during the entire procedure and can go home the same day or the next morning. Convalescence is very short (about one week).

Cardiac surgery (bypasses), on the other hand, obviously requires general anaesthetic. Most of the time, a special solution is used to stop the heart from beating (cardioplegia) and blood circulation is ensured using a device commonly called a *heart-lung machine* or, more scientifically, a *cardiopulmonary bypass machine* (*CPB*). The blood is thus channelled to a device that replaces the functions of the heart and

BALLOON AND STENT ANGIOPLASTY

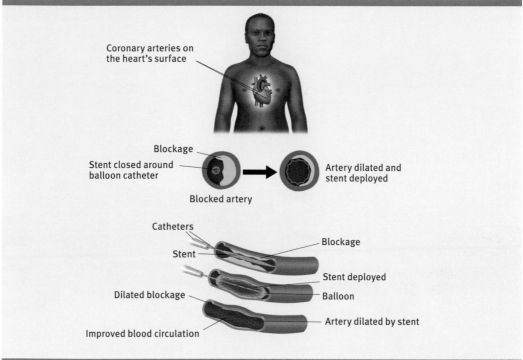

FIGURE 13

lungs, supplying the blood with oxygen and then returning it to the body. This device is operated by a very specialized technician called a *perfusionist*. The surgery lasts about three hours and requires a much longer convalescence (from one to three months).

LONG-TERM TREATMENT AFTER ANGIOPLASTY AND CARDIAC SURGERY

Balloon angioplasty and coronary artery bypass surgery do not cure the patient. These operations are very effective in reducing angina pain. Patients must nonetheless be reminded that the conditions that caused a blockage in their coronary arteries are still there and that they can again "attack"

arteries unblocked by balloons or bypasses. If patients do not change their lifestyle and do not take the effective medications recommended, the symptoms will recur and everything will have to be done again. Unfortunately, this is what often happens with many people who feel completely cured. We must therefore ensure that a patient who has undergone one of these operations follows what we call a *secondary* prevention program, also known as *cardiac rehabilitation*.

TREATING AN ACUTE HEART ATTACK OR UNSTABLE ANGINA

In the case of a heart attack or unstable angina (very severe angina that quickly

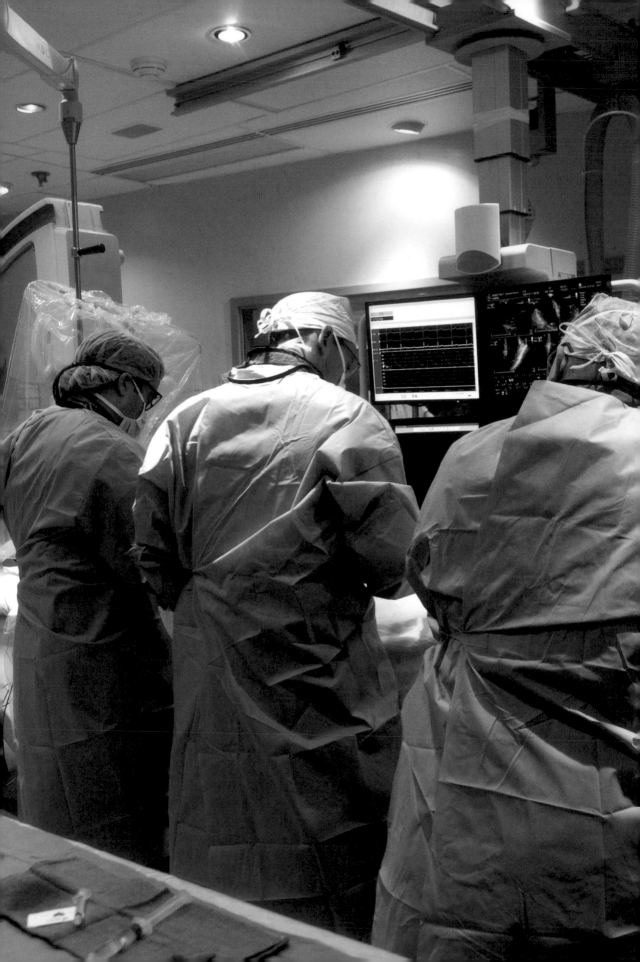

CORONARY ARTERY BYPASSES

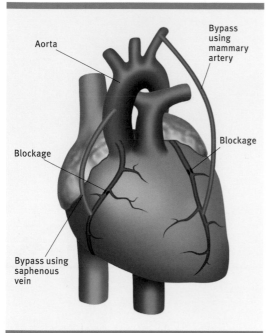

Aorta

Bypass using mammary artery

Blockage

Blockage

Bypass using saphenous vein

FIGURE 14

leads to a heart attack if it's not treated), aggressive treatment is immediately needed. During an acute heart attack, the coronary artery is completely blocked by a clot. The patient must therefore be admitted as quickly as possible to a cardiac catheterization room for an angioplasty (in this case called primary angioplasty). A

guide is threaded into and across the entire blockage, a balloon is inserted to dilate the blockage, and a stent is left in place. In most cases, the developing heart attack can be stopped. The faster this treatment is given, the less damage there will be to the heart muscle: every minute counts (in cardiology we say, "Time is muscle," referring to the financial dictum "Time is money"). Medical teams are actually evaluated according to how fast they act; in other words, the number of minutes that elapse between the admission of the patient at the hospital door and the opening of the blocked artery is calculated ("door-to-balloon time").

We regularly see patients arrive an hour after the intense pain caused by a heart attack has begun. The artery is then immediately dilated, and patients are discharged less than thirty-six hours later. They usually have very few after effects. Conversely, if the patient puts off going to emergency and the pain lasts more than six hours, the damage is much greater. In short, during a heart attack or unstable angina, 911 must be called quickly. Rapid intervention can save the patient's life and minimize the after effects.

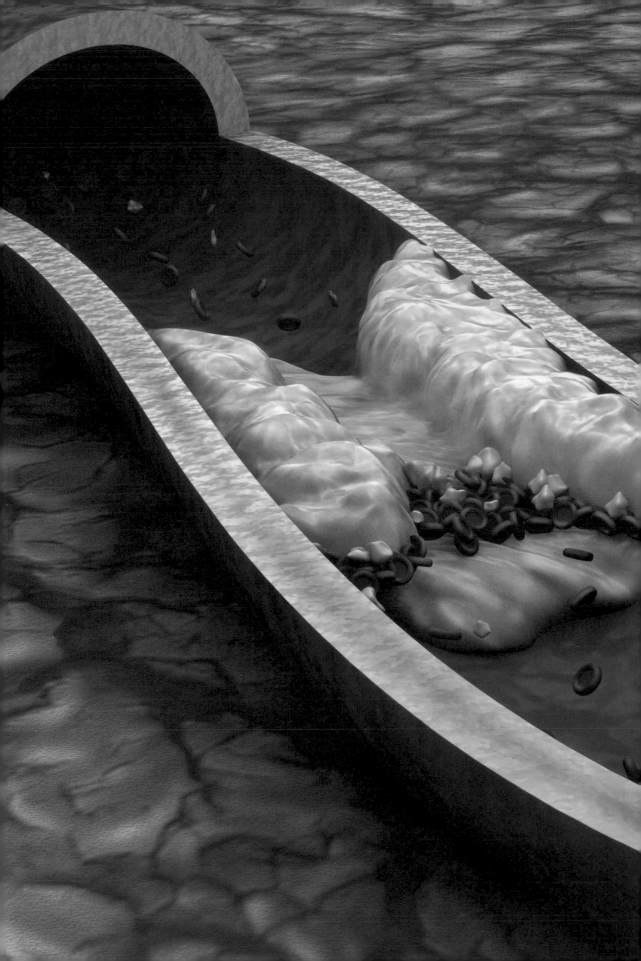

CHAPTER 3

At the Heart of the Problem: Atherosclerosis

As the name indicates, cardiovascular disease includes all diseases of the heart and blood vessels. However, the cardiovascular disease that causes heart attacks and angina, and results in the most sudden deaths, is *coronary heart disease*, which attacks the coronary arteries supplying the heart muscle. This disease is in turn caused by atherosclerosis. More than just "traffic jams" that deprive the heart of the oxygen it needs to function, atherosclerotic plaques are in fact the result of a very complex process involving a wide range of biochemical, immune-related, genetic, and epigenetic factors. Averting or at the very least slowing down the development of the process of atherosclerosis is therefore absolutely indispensable for preventing cardiovascular disease.

AN INFLAMMATORY DISEASE

Atherosclerosis is a chronic disease of the arterial lining that develops silently over many years, without causing any visible symptoms. The interior wall of the arteries is covered by a thin layer of what are called *endothelial cells*, or *endothelium*. Very important for vascular health, the endothelium is found in all the body's arteries, from the largest to the smallest capillary vessels. It's the first line of defence against various "attacks": inflammation, viruses, bacteria, high cholesterol levels, toxic products in cigarette smoke, etc. If the endothelium suffers too many attacks, it can no longer play its protective role, allowing atherosclerosis to take hold gradually. Initially, the plaques are just fat deposits smeared

DEVELOPMENT OF ATHEROSCLEROSIS

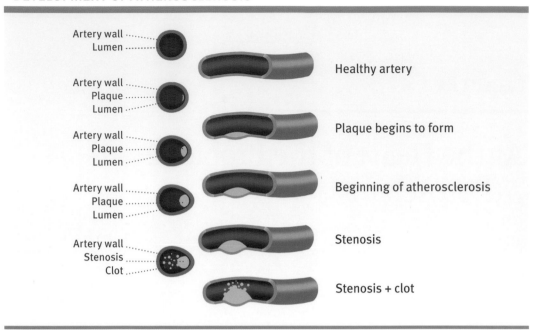

Artery wall
Lumen
Healthy artery

Artery wall
Plaque
Lumen
Plaque begins to form

Artery wall
Plaque
Lumen
Beginning of atherosclerosis

Artery wall
Plaque
Lumen
Stenosis

Artery wall
Stenosis
Clot
Stenosis + clot

FIGURE 15

along the artery's interior lining, *fatty streaks* caused by the infiltration of certain white blood cells that store cholesterol and cause the plaque to accumulate in the vessel's muscle wall (Figure 15). This causes a chronic local inflammatory reaction that, through a series of complex events, stimulates the growth of muscle cells in the vessel wall, and triggers the formation of a fibrous layer that separates the immune cells and fatty substances from the bloodstream. When they remain in this form, these plaques pose no immediate danger to health, since the fibrous layer is quite stable and manages to hermetically seal off the fatty deposits in the artery wall. The arteries also have enough elasticity to stretch so as to retain their normal diameter and maintain the same rate of blood flow despite the presence of plaques (the Glagov phenomenon). On the other hand, when the volume of the atherosclerotic plaque becomes too great, the partial blockage of the vessel causes a reduction in the blood reaching the heart muscle. This partial blockage may typically manifest itself as pain during exertion (angina).

Often, however, vessel blockage resulting in a heart attack is not caused by a large plaque blocking blood circulation but instead by a clot (a thrombus) formed from much smaller plaques. These rupturing plaques are a result of uncontrolled chronic inflammation in the artery wall: the death of too many cells in the centre of the plaque destabilizes the fibrous layer, triggering the development of very thin and fragile areas on the plaque's surface. The rupture or erosion of these plaques exposes their contents to the clotting system, which, believing this

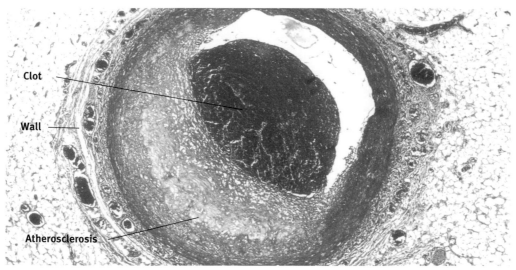

Clot

Wall

Atherosclerosis

↗ Section of a blocked artery seen under a microscope.

is an injury in need of repair, immediately forms a clot that completely blocks the vessel. This is a very dangerous situation, as there will be few symptoms, and sometimes none at all, to alert us to the sudden blockage. Indeed, as was mentioned in the preceding chapter, sudden death is often the first sign of atherosclerosis, which accounts for 50% of deaths from cardiovascular disease in our societies.

INNATE PREDISPOSITION

Atherosclerosis is not a recent disorder: the analysis of Egyptian mummies has revealed calcifications in the blood vessels of almost half the deceased, including severe atherosclerosis affecting the entire arterial network of a princess who lived around 1600 BCE. Similar observations have been made with respect to the mummified bodies of Peruvians, Anasazis (Indigenous peoples from southwestern North America), and Aleuts (Alaskan Inuit) dating from about one thousand years ago. Most of these individuals were quite young when they died (43 years old on average) and lived well before the industrial era but several thousand years after the emergence of agriculture and livestock farming, suggesting that their diet could in some ways have resembled our own.

The appearance of coronary atherosclerosis at a very young age is clearly illustrated in the results of autopsies on young adults who died of causes other than cardiovascular disease. During the Korean War, for example, 77% of the autopsies of American soldiers, on average 22 years old and killed in battle, revealed the presence of atherosclerotic plaques, as well as the complete obstruction of one or more vessels in 3% of these individuals. Premature atherosclerosis has also been observed in soldiers who fought in Vietnam, as well as in children and young adults living in many parts of the world. This early onset has been especially well documented in Bogalusa (in the state of Louisiana), where a study done on children and adults who died young (of causes unrelated to heart diseases) showed that the first stages of atherosclerosis (fatty streaks and fibrous plaques) appeared very early in life, both in the aorta and in the coronary arteries (Figure 16). In some extreme cases (maternal hypercholesterolemia), these plaques could even be detected before birth in the fetus's arterial network!

The PDAY Study, conducted worldwide, confirmed these observations and showed that atherosclerotic plaques in the aorta are found in a significant proportion of individuals aged 15 to 19. Almost half of these adolescents also have plaques in their coronary arteries, a proportion that increases steadily in later decades, with more than 70% of individuals in their forties affected. These observations confirm that atherosclerotic plaques appear very early in life, regardless of sex, race, or geographic origin.

In short, a heart attack occurring in adulthood is the end of a long process in which the first fatty deposits appear in childhood and gradually evolve into fibrous plaques with the potential to obstruct blood circulation (Figure 17).

This innate predisposition to atherosclerosis therefore means that we are all at risk for cardiovascular disease. It also explains why heart diseases are such a major cause of mortality in the population. Yet why are some people struck down by these diseases in the prime of life, while others, on the contrary, reach old age without ever being affected? In other words, what are the factors that can influence to this extent the development of atherosclerosis and cardiovascular disease?

PREVALENCE OF ATHEROSCLEROTIC PLAQUES IN THE AORTAS AND CORONARY ARTERIES OF CHILDREN AND YOUNG ADULTS

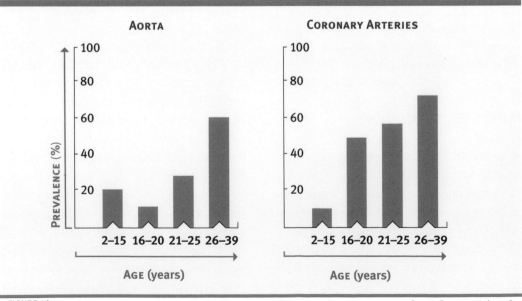

FIGURE 16   Source: Berenson et al., 1998

RISK FACTORS

A vast number of studies done in the last seventy-five years have allowed us to better understand these risk factors. First, there are what are called non-modifiable risk factors, those beyond our control:

- age, because the spontaneous formation of atheromatous plaques throughout our lifetime means that these plaques cover more and more of the surface of our blood vessels as we age, increasing the risk of obstruction;

- sex, because women are affected by cardiovascular disease on average ten years later than men (owing to the protection offered by estrogens); and

- heredity, because we do not choose our parents and some families are at greater risk by virtue of certain genetic variations that promote the atherosclerotic process.

ATHEROSCLEROSIS: A CHRONIC DISEASE THAT BEGINS IN CHILDHOOD

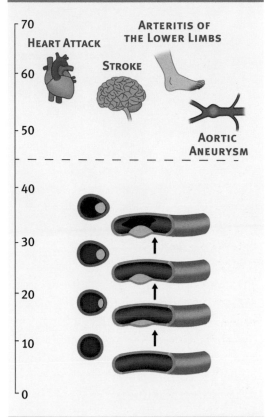

FIGURE 17   Source: Adapted from McGill et al., 2000

Overall, it's estimated that these non-modifiable risk factors are responsible for 15% to 20% of deaths associated with coronary diseases, a much lower proportion than that of deaths caused by a series of modifiable factors, directly related to lifestyle (Figure 18). Bad diet, lack of physical activity, smoking, and too much stress are the four *primordial* factors that increase mortality risk, since they cause many metabolic disturbances like obesity, high blood pressure, and insulin resistance (hyperglycemia).

The importance of these modifiable factors is clearly shown by the dramatic variations in the incidence of cardiovascular disease worldwide, as well as among migrant populations. For example, whereas Japan has one of the lowest incidences of cardiovascular diseases in the world, this number doubles among Japanese who immigrate to Hawaii and quadruples among those who choose to live in San Francisco (Figure 19). What is surprising is that this increase does not depend on blood pressure or cholesterol level, but rather seems to be directly related to the migrants' abandonment of a traditional Japanese way of life. In other words, even though these Japanese have

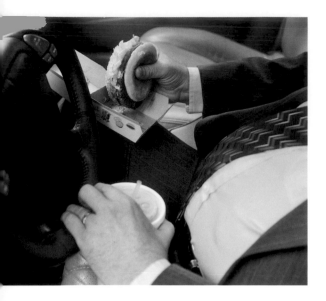

the same non-modifiable risk factors (age, sex, and heredity) as their fellow Japanese remaining in their country of birth, the simple fact that they adopt the lifestyle habits of their country of destination is enough to considerably increase their risk of cardiovascular disease.

TARGETS FOR PREVENTION

The prevention of cardiovascular disease is therefore, in theory, relatively simple: first, it's a matter of modifying the pri-mordial risk factors (diet, physical activity, smoking, and stress), so as to reduce the negative impact of the obesity, high blood pressure, and high blood sugar they cause. A good example of the benefits of *primor-dial* prevention is the rate of smoking: the many anti-tobacco campaigns, higher taxes, and bans on smoking in public places have resulted in a significant decrease in smoking in recent decades, which has led to a considerable decrease

Three Levels of Prevention

Primordial Prevention

This tries, at very early stages, even before the risk factor appears, to prevent activities that encourage the emergence of lifestyles, behaviours, and harmful influences that contribute to a high rate of disease. For example, a child who sees his parents smoking might conclude, wrongly, that this is a good lifestyle choice. In this situation, advising parents to stop smoking would be an example of primordial prevention.

Primary Prevention

This is a matter of preventing disease by trying to control exposure to risk fac-tors. For example, keeping a watchful eye on your weight and especially on your waist circumference prevents abdo-minal obesity, which is also a risk factor for a number of ailments, including heart disease and diabetes.

Secondary Prevention

In cardiology, the term "secondary preven-tion" is used to describe an intervention aiming to avoid the adverse progression of an already established disease and, thus, to prevent it from getting worse or recurring.

in the number of cases of cardiovascular disease and lung cancer (see Chapter 8).

Oddly, a prevention strategy based on primordial factors has not been applied systematically or aggressively. For example,

MAIN RISK FACTORS FOR HEART DISEASE

Non-Modifiable		Modifiable	
		Primordial	Traditional
Age		Smoking	High LDL cholesterol
Sex	**+**	Diet	Low HDL cholesterol
Heredity		Physical activity	High blood pressure
		Stress	Obesity
			High blood sugar
			Metabolic syndrome

FIGURE 18

even though it's known that a bad diet and a sedentary lifestyle are the *primary causes* of a large proportion of cardiovascular diseases, it's instead the *consequences* of these bad habits (high blood pressure, high cholesterol, or high blood sugar) that are targeted by the classic medical approach. So, if your blood test indicates you have a higher than normal level of LDL cholesterol, it's customary to immediately prescribe anti-cholesterol (statin) or high blood pressure medication. Rarely do we try to correct these anomalies *at the source*, by recommending instead a change in diet and regular physical exercise. In a recent editorial, Dr. Dariush Mozaffarian, dean of the Friedman School of Nutrition Science and Policy at Tufts University in Boston, summarized the approach that should be emphasized this way: "For both individual patients and populations, lifestyle goals should not be formulated solely for control of weight or blood pressure, cholesterol, and glucose levels. Although lifestyle has major benefits on these physiological factors, a healthier diet, greater activity, and nonsmoking influence numerous other pathways of risk and produce substantial additional benefits for cardiovascular and noncardiovascular health." Dr. Mozaffarian concludes that "patients should enter their doctor's office and not simply ask 'How are my blood pressure, cholesterol, and glucose levels?' but also ask 'How are my dietary habits, physical activity level, smoking, and waist measurement?'"

The importance of targeting the primordial causes of cardiovascular disease (diet, activity, smoking, stress) in order to effectively prevent it will be discussed in detail in the chapters that follow. Before looking at these aspects, however, we need to understand the reasons why the medical community has, for forty years, been in the habit of tackling the effects instead of the causes of these disorders, as well as the limits of this approach.

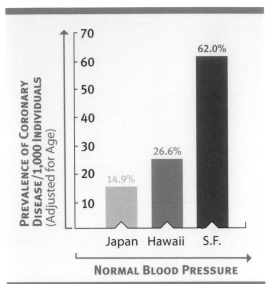

PREVALENCE OF CORONARY DISEASE AMONG JAPANESE LIVING IN JAPAN, HAWAII, AND SAN FRANCISCO

FIGURE 19   Source: Marmot et al., 1975

CHOLESTEROL

Few substances have left as much of a mark on the history of the sciences as cholesterol: no fewer than thirteen Nobel Prize winners have dedicated their research work to this molecule. This is a legitimate interest, since cholesterol plays an extremely important role in the functioning of the human body, both as a component of cell membranes and as a basic ingredient in the production of a number of essential substances, like bile salts and certain vitamins (vitamin D), as well as several hormones (sex hormones, corticoids, etc.).

Mainly produced in the liver, cholesterol is insoluble in water (and therefore in the bloodstream) and must use a transport system that is adapted for the purpose of reaching different cells in the organism.

Low-density lipoproteins (LDL) transport cholesterol from the liver to the cells, while high-density lipoproteins (HDL) do the opposite — they capture the excess cholesterol and take it back to the liver, where it will be eliminated (Figure 20).

A great many studies have established that anomalies in the blood levels of these two types of cholesterol have a major influence on the risk of coronary disease. Too much LDL cholesterol, for example, means that a larger amount of cholesterol comes into contact with the artery walls, which can then accelerate the formation of atheromatous plaques. The result is a considerable increase in the risk of cardiovascular problems in people with high levels of LDL cholesterol — hence its name "bad cholesterol" (Figure 21).

This connection is especially well documented in people with familial hypercholesterolemia (FH), a genetic disorder that exposes individuals to high levels of LDL cholesterol from birth, owing to an inability to properly eliminate it. If they are not treated, people with heterozygous FH (transmission of the defective gene by a single parent) run the risk of having a coronary event before age 55, whereas those with homozygous FH (transmission of the defective gene by both parents) can die before even reaching adulthood. Worldwide, it's thought that roughly one person in five hundred has FH, but this prevalence is much higher in some regions, in particular in northeastern Quebec (Côte-Nord, Lac Saint-Jean), where it may affect at least one in every one hundred people.

There is also a link between HDL cholesterol levels and the risk of coronary disease, but this time in reverse — high levels promote the elimination of cholesterol and are therefore beneficial for heart health, hence its name "good" cholesterol.

It's because of all this well-known data that measuring LDL and HDL cholesterol levels has been included in basic blood testing for more than thirty years, and that any deviation from normal values is considered to be a risk factor for coronary disease.

It's important to understand, however, that a high LDL cholesterol level is not a disease in itself but really a *risk factor* for coronary disease. Cholesterol level must therefore be considered as one element in a complex whole, taking into account lifestyle habits and all the other risk factors.

HIGH BLOOD PRESSURE

Affecting over one billion people worldwide, high blood pressure is directly responsible for nearly ten million deaths every year, making it the biggest risk factor for premature death worldwide. The major impact of blood pressure that is too high is to cause, over time, a thickening and hardening of the arteries, mechanical stress that promotes the development of atherosclerosis, as well as the rupture of atheromatous plaques. Several studies have shown that there is a close relationship between blood pressure above the normal level (higher than 115/75 mm Hg) and the risk of coronary events or stroke, at every age and in all demographic groups. Controlling blood pressure is thus essential in preventing cardiovascular disease. This explains why anti-hypertensives are the most prescribed drugs in Canada, just ahead of drugs that treat high cholesterol.

Studies prove that these medications reduce the risk of coronary disease (by 15% to 25%), stroke (by 35% to 40%) and heart failure (by up to 65%). It appears, however, that these medications are most beneficial for hypertensive people whose systolic pressure is higher than 160 mm Hg. If they are given to people whose pressure is higher than normal, but not at that high a level, a real, but more modest, reduction in risk of death from heart disease is

↗ Cholesterol molecule

CHOLESTEROL TRANSPORT IN THE BODY (SIMPLIFIED)

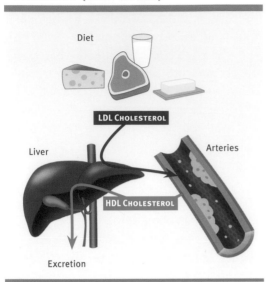

FIGURE 20

observed. Patients treated successfully with anti-hypertensive drugs still have a 2.5 times higher risk of having a heart attack than people who are naturally normotensive (whose blood pressure is normal with no pharmacological treatment) with the same blood pressure. It's therefore more effective for health to treat the *causes* of high blood pressure — poor diet, obesity, and sedentariness — rather than opting for a drug. That said, if you cannot manage to lower your blood pressure by changing your lifestyle habits, you should not hesitate to take the medications prescribed by your doctor. Untreated high blood pressure can cause very serious damage to the kidneys, retina, brain, and, obviously, heart.

High blood pressure rarely develops in isolation, and this is one of the factors limiting the benefits of anti-hypertensive drugs. Hypertensive people very often have other "classic" risk factors for cardiovascular

disease, such as being overweight or obese (especially in the abdomen) and having overly high blood lipid levels (dyslipidemia) or sugar metabolism disorders (insulin resistance). Given the rapid rise in recent decades of obesity and the number of people who are overweight, it's more and more common for an individual to be affected by several of these factors. This is known as "metabolic syndrome."

METABOLIC SYNDROME

Metabolic syndrome is not a disease in the strict sense of the term but a cluster of a number of metabolic disorders that, taken together, greatly increase the risk of cardiovascular diseases (Figure 22):

- large waist circumference (>102 centimetres [41 inches] for men and > 88 centimetres [35 inches] for women
- hypertriglyceridemia (>1.7 mmol/L)
- low HDL cholesterol (<1.0 mmol/L for men and <1.3 mmol/L for women)
- high fasting glucose level (> 6.1 mmol/L, or taking hypoglycemic medication)
- hypertension (>135/85 mm Hg, or taking anti-hypertensive medication)

People with one or two of these disorders have twice the risk of being prematurely affected by cardiovascular disease; in individuals with all these conditions who also have diabetes, the risk can be as much as five times as high.

The work of Dr. Jean-Pierre Després at Laval University has clearly established that too much abdominal fat is a greater

INCIDENCE OF MORTALITY ASSOCIATED WITH CORONARY DISEASE AS A FUNCTION OF CHOLESTEROL LEVEL, ACCORDING TO THE MRFIT STUDY

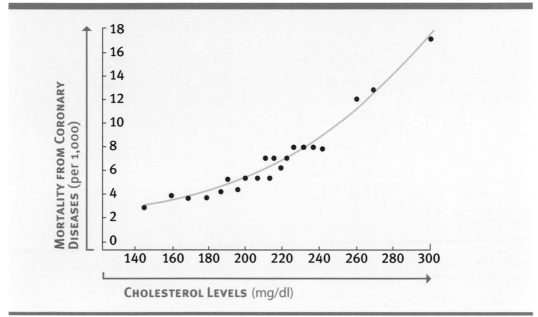

FIGURE 21

Source: Martin et al., 1986

risk factor for cardiovascular disease than fat located in other parts of the body — on the hips, for example. One of the most damaging impacts of this excess abdominal fat is to reduce the effectiveness of insulin in stimulating the absorption of sugar by some organs, especially the muscles, liver, and adipose tissue. This *insulin resistance* means that the amount of sugar in the blood remains too high (clinically measured by a higher than normal fasting glucose level), forcing the pancreas to secrete even more insulin so that sugar can enter the cells. When this goes on for too long, insulin resistance can cause pancreatic exhaustion, resulting in the onset of type 2 diabetes.

In terms of cardiovascular disease, the onset of type 2 diabetes is nothing less than a catastrophe; people with chronic high blood pressure have a very high risk of having a coronary event, along with a whole range of complications. Furthermore, this condition is extremely difficult to treat with drugs. The medications used up to now to treat type 2 diabetes have little or no effect in terms of reducing cardiovascular disease risk and can have major side effects that negatively impact patients' quality of life.

In summary, the current medical approach for preventing cardiovascular diseases essentially consists of taking control of high cholesterol, high blood pressure, and high blood sugar by means of drugs. This strategy may seem effective on the surface, since medications do indeed manage to normalize cholesterol, blood pressure, and blood sugar in most patients, which may lead us to believe that the situation is under control and the risk of having a heart attack or stroke has been eliminated. Unfortunately, this is not the case: many studies have indicated that maintaining a normal cholesterol level

The Limits of the Risk Score

Let's take the example of a 63-year-old man who has no family history of heart disease, is vegetarian, does thirty minutes of exercise a day, maintains a healthy weight, has a waist circumference of 81 cm, systolic blood pressure of 130 mm Hg, a total cholesterol level of 5.2 mmol/L, and an HDL level of 1.25 mmol/L. According to the Framingham risk scale, this man's risk of developing heart disease in the next ten years is 18.4%, a moderately high percentage. Many doctors will therefore recommend he take a statin, which is absurd, since in reality the risk of this man's having a heart attack is almost zero. Conversely, a 38-year-old man who is obese and sedentary, smokes twenty-five cigarettes a day, eats junk food, and has the same numbers for cholesterol and blood pressure (because the numbers have not yet begun to rise at this age) will be considered low risk (9.4%), whereas he is, in fact, a walking time bomb: heart attack, sudden death, and stroke are lying in wait for him. These examples are not theoretical: I see variations on these two typical cases every week in my practice at the EPIC Centre. Furthermore, I know the first case very well: it's me.

by means of pharmacological intervention (statins) reduces the absolute risk of coronary disease only by about 1% (see Chapter 9). The same is true of high blood sugar medication: these drugs can help control blood sugar levels in the short and medium term, but if the patient remains sedentary and carries too much weight, they cannot halt the progression of atherosclerosis.

Atherosclerosis is a very complex multi-factorial process and no medication, no matter how effective, can fix all the health problems associated with poor lifestyle habits, such as a diet low in nutrients and sedentariness, on its own. In other words, the protection drugs offer should not be discounted, but we can do much better by attacking the root causes underlying the development of cardiovascular disease.

This is as true for preventing a first heart attack as for improving quality of life for people who have already experienced a coronary event. For example, a study done by Canadian cardiologist Salim Yusuf showed that patients who change their diet and follow a regular exercise program after a heart attack see their risk of recurrence cut in half compared with those who do not change their habits (Figure 23). Since all these patients were treated with all the usual drugs (beta-blockers, statins, Aspirin, etc.), these results show just how much lifestyle can influence the risk of recurrence.

Changing our approach to preventing cardiovascular disease is therefore desirable. Routinely, in medicine, the risk of having a coronary event is estimated based essentially on age and on a series of quantifiable measurements (cholesterol, blood sugar, and blood pressure), but without taking into account dietary habits, physical activity level, and waist circumference. These three factors are not even part of the "risk scores" used in clinical practice. The Framingham

METABOLIC SYNDROME

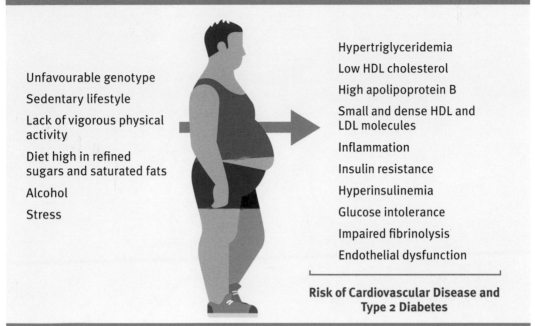

Unfavourable genotype

Sedentary lifestyle

Lack of vigorous physical activity

Diet high in refined sugars and saturated fats

Alcohol

Stress

Hypertriglyceridemia

Low HDL cholesterol

High apolipoprotein B

Small and dense HDL and LDL molecules

Inflammation

Insulin resistance

Hyperinsulinemia

Glucose intolerance

Impaired fibrinolysis

Endothelial dysfunction

Risk of Cardiovascular Disease and Type 2 Diabetes

FIGURE 22   Adapted from Després, 2015

score, for example, the best known and most used, ignores these factors.

Tackling a single target, like blood pressure or cholesterol level, is of course much easier than taking aim at all of the factors responsible for the progression of a disease as complex as atherosclerosis. No drug, however, no matter how effective it may be in correcting the imbalances caused by a poor diet and a sedentary lifestyle, will be able to provide the same benefits as a preventive approach that tackles the *source* of the problems. In clinical practice, we must provide patients with all the information they need and give them the choice: we call this a "patient-partner approach."

The goal of the chapters that follow is precisely to make the scientific data currently available on the factors that influence the risk of cardiovascular disease better known.

EFFECT OF DIET AND EXERCISE ON MORTALITY RISK IN PATIENTS WHO HAVE HAD A CORONARY EVENT

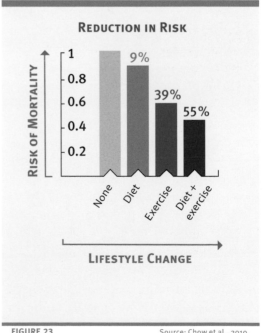

REDUCTION IN RISK

FIGURE 23   Source: Chow et al., 2010.

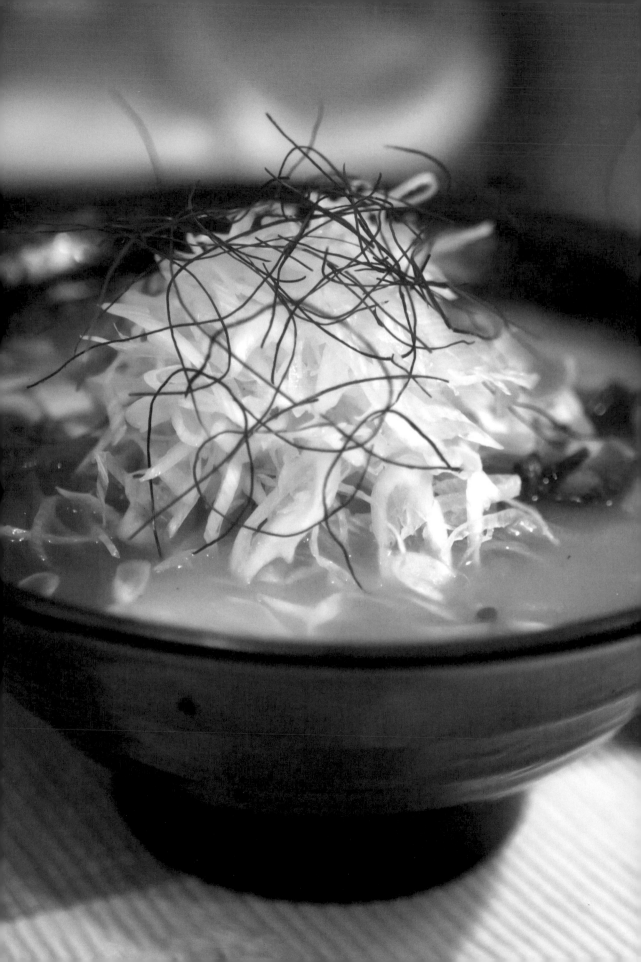

CHAPTER 4

Diet and Cardiovascular Disease

A high-quality diet is one of the main pillars of chronic disease prevention and the maintenance of good health in general. Yet despite its importance, there still exists a great deal of confusion about what a "healthy" diet really is. Every day, I hear my patients complain that nutritional recommendations keep changing, that what is good one day is not good the next (or the opposite), and that, as a result, "we just don't know what to eat anymore."

This frustration over diet is, to some extent, understandable, for never before have we had access to so much information about the contents of our daily foods. Modern nutrition has become a very complicated science for the average person!

The situation becomes even more complex when studies that examine the impact of these various elements on health reach contradictory conclusions. In cardiology, the best example is undoubtedly the influence of saturated fats on heart attack risk. Many studies have shown that replacing saturated fats with polyunsaturated (omega-3) or monounsaturated vegetable fats reduces the risk of heart attack. This is why for many years replacing butter with vegetable oils, like olive or canola oil, has been recommended. On the other hand, a number of recent analyses have not found a link between consuming saturated fats and cardiovascular disease risk: this was all it took for the media to seize on the information and proclaim that "Butter is Back," a *Time Magazine* headline in 2014. This enthusiasm was, however, unfounded, as we will see later, and only added to consumers' confusion.

In fact, the situation is much simpler than we might think. Instead of dwelling too much on the results of studies examining a very precise class of nutrients (saturated fats, for example), it's much more useful to examine dietary habits *overall*. Individuals do not eat just one type of nutrient, but rather a range of foods at meals, containing many elements that will interact with each other and mutually influence their impact on the human body. And only when people's dietary habits are observed as a whole can we see that eating well is really not all that complicated.

THE HEALTHY EATING PLATE

The main principles of a healthy diet have been known for many years, thanks especially to the work of experts in nutrition and preventive medicine, like Walter Willett and David Ludwig of Harvard University and David Katz of Yale University. These principles, recently confirmed in a report of more than five hundred pages produced by a group of specialists consulted by the United States Department of Agriculture (USDA), are illustrated in "the healthy eating plate" (Figure 24).

In practical terms, in a healthy diet, lots of room is reserved for plant foods (like fruits, vegetables, legumes, and whole-grain cereals), the consumption of animal products is reduced (red meat, for example), and processed industrial foods are avoided as much as possible (processed meats, sugary drinks, and junk food). A healthy diet includes a high intake of complex carbohydrates (fibre and whole grains, for example) and a moderate amount of protein, derived mainly from plants, fish, or poultry. In addition, the recommended fats are mainly *unsaturated* (including a large proportion of omega-3) rather than saturated. While not at all revolutionary, this combination is nonetheless optimal

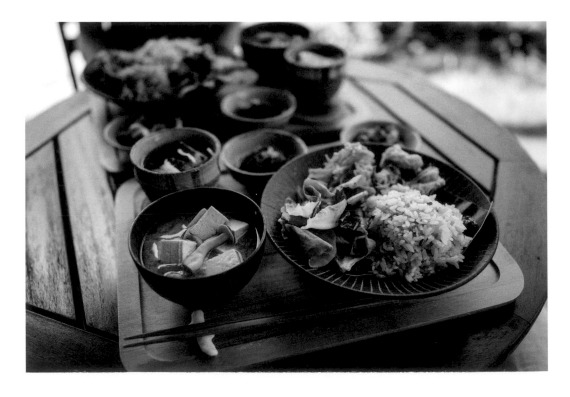

THE HARVARD UNIVERSITY SCHOOL OF PUBLIC HEALTH HEALTHY EATING PLATE

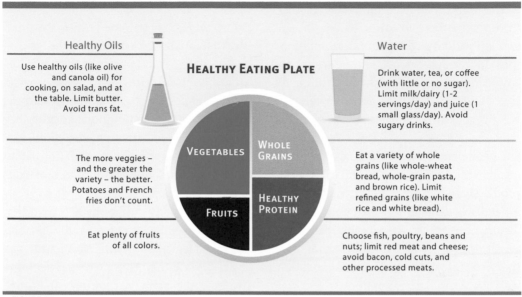

Healthy Oils

Use healthy oils (like olive and canola oil) for cooking, on salad, and at the table. Limit butter. Avoid trans fat.

HEALTHY EATING PLATE

Water

Drink water, tea, or coffee (with little or no sugar). Limit milk/dairy (1-2 servings/day) and juice (1 small glass/day). Avoid sugary drinks.

The more veggies – and the greater the variety – the better. Potatoes and French fries don't count.

VEGETABLES

WHOLE GRAINS

Eat a variety of whole grains (like whole-wheat bread, whole-grain pasta, and brown rice). Limit refined grains (like white rice and white bread).

FRUITS

HEALTHY PROTEIN

Eat plenty of fruits of all colors.

Choose fish, poultry, beans and nuts; limit red meat and cheese; avoid bacon, cold cuts, and other processed meats.

FIGURE 24

for health, as the predominance of plants results in a high intake of nutrients and antioxidant and anti-inflammatory compounds. This diet also ensures that too sudden blood sugar fluctuations and the excess calories associated with consuming animal and processed products are avoided.

These principles can be summarized by the famous dictum of American journalist Michael Pollan, an expert analyst of modern dietary habits, who says, "Eat food, not too much, mostly plants." He adds, "And nothing that your great-grandmother would not recognize as food."

By "eat food," Michael Pollan means that we should eat "real" food, whole and fresh, rather than processed foods to which all kinds of products more or less harmful to health have been added. "Not too much" obviously means that we should consume fewer calories. "Mostly plants" emphasizes that most of our calories should come from plant sources (fruits, vegetables, legumes, nuts) rather than animal sources. "And nothing that your great-grandmother would not recognize as food" of course refers to the ultra-processed products manufactured by the food industry.

Eating well to live a long and healthy life is extremely simple. It's a matter of adopting a semi-vegetarian diet, as is already the case in parts of the world where the most exceptional longevity is observed: the island of Okinawa in Japan, some parts of Sardinia, the Nicoya peninsula in Costa Rica, the island of Ikaria in Greece, and the city of Loma Linda in California. Journalist Dan Buettner has published three books in which he describes the way of life in these areas, which he has dubbed "Blue Zones."

The principles of a healthy diet are, however, diametrically opposed to modern dietary habits, in particular those of the inhabitants of industrialized countries. There is no doubt that this is what contributes to the high incidence of chronic diseases in our societies. Not only do we not eat enough plant-based foods, but, in addition, most of our daily calories come from processed industrial food products. It's thought that currently about 60% of the calories we ingest come from these kinds of foods, made from low-quality, cheap ingredients, and engineered first and foremost to satisfy our cravings for fat, sugar, and salt. These products are harmful to health, since they are usually lacking in essential nutrients like dietary fibre, and contain on the other hand astronomical amounts of fat, sugar, and therefore calories, which causes too much weight gain and inflammation.

In terms of preventing chronic diseases, the most important point is therefore to fix this imbalance by increasing plant intake. This is not just because this change is of necessity, accompanied by a reduction in processed foods, but also because this simple change alone will influence the kind of protein, carbohydrates, and lipids ingested, as well as, at the same time, all of the processes that favour the onset and progression of atherosclerotic plaques. In the pages that follow, curious readers will be able to familiarize themselves with the scientific data underlying these recommendations. On the other hand, those with less time who want to immediately understand the impact of a diet higher in plant-based products on risk reduction for cardiovascular disease can consult Chapter 5, where the practical applications of these recommendations are discussed — in other words, the Mediterranean diet, as well as vegetarian and vegan diets.

PLANT PROTECTION

Worldwide, it's estimated that 2.2 million deaths caused by coronary disease and strokes are directly related to the inadequate consumption of fruits and vegetables. Yet despite many campaigns aiming to promote the consumption of plants, they remain the poor cousins of current dietary habits: barely 20% of the population eats at least five daily servings (400 grams) of fruits and vegetables per day.

A great many studies have shown that people who eat a lot of fruit and vegetables are much less likely to suffer from cardiovascular disease than those who eat very few. For example, a major study done in Europe (EPIC-Heart Study) among 313,074 men and women in good health revealed that people who ate at least eight servings of fruits and vegetables a day had a 22% lower risk of dying prematurely from a coronary disease, compared with those who ate three servings or fewer. Both classes of plants seem to be necessary to cause this protective effect: for example, even though the Chinese regularly eat a lot of fresh vegetables, one study recently showed that those who ate in addition one piece of fruit a day saw their risk of cardiovascular disease decrease by 40%. Overall, studies indicate that each serving of fruit and vegetables reduces the risk of cardiovascular disease by 4%, showing just how important it is to incorporate these plants into our dietary habits.

Several factors have been suggested to explain the positive impact of fruits and vegetables on the risk of cardiovascular disease (Figure 25). It appears, however, that it's the combination of all these elements that is responsible for the benefits associated with eating these foods. For

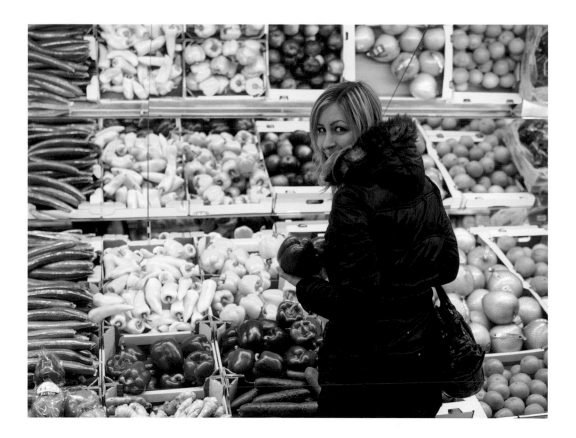

example, although it's undeniable that plants' high vitamin and mineral content influences levels of inflammation and oxidative stress, both of which contribute to the process of atherosclerosis, no study has been able to demonstrate that *supplements* containing high amounts of these elements could lower mortality risk from cardiovascular disease. There is nothing surprising in this, since fruits and vegetables contain many other bioactive molecules, such as polyphenols, in the flavonoid class, that can also influence the atherosclerotic process. In other words, no purified molecule can replace the molecular complexity of plants. The only way to get the most benefit from these foods is to incorporate them into our dietary habits.

MAIN BENEFICIAL EFFECTS OF FRUITS AND VEGETABLES ON CARDIOVASCULAR HEALTH

Fruits and vegetables are
- anti-hypertensive;
- antioxidant; and
- anti-inflammatory.

In addition, these plants
- normalize blood lipid levels;
- modify the intestinal biome;
- improve blood sugar control; and
- have low caloric density.

FIGURE 25

Although it's never too late, the ideal is to begin eating fruits and vegetables in childhood, as a lower incidence of coronary artery calcification (a well-established indicator of atherosclerosis) has been noted in people who consume a lot of plant foods early in adulthood than in those who begin to eat them later in life. Unfortunately, only 10% of Canadian children ages 12 to 17 eat the minimum recommended amount of fruits and vegetables. As a result, they are likely to develop cardiovascular disease at some point in their lives.

CEREAL GRAINS: THE IMPORTANCE OF WHOLE GRAINS

The carbohydrates in the modern diet also contribute to the epidemics of obesity and chronic diseases, including cardiovascular diseases, currently sweeping the planet. A great many of the products consumed daily are made from white refined flours (bread, pasta, baked goods, etc.) or contain large amounts of added sugars (soft drinks and junk food in general). This is a troubling situation, since when sugar is consumed in these forms it's very quickly assimilated by the intestine and causes a rapid surge in blood sugar on reaching the bloodstream. Our metabolism is poorly adapted to these sudden fluctuations in sugar, which over time cause a number of metabolic upheavals with serious repercussions for the development of atherosclerosis.

Studies in recent years have shown that the simple sugars (as opposed to complex sugars) that are added to a wide range of processed products, especially soft drinks and various snack foods (Figure 26), are especially harmful to health. People who

SOURCES OF ADDED SUGARS IN FOODS

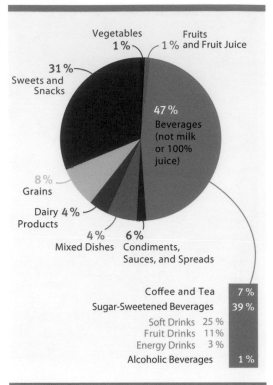

FIGURE 26 Source: Adapted from Mitka, 2006
* Totals do not add to 100% because of rounding

frequently consume foods containing these added sugars have a higher risk of obesity, type 2 diabetes, and cardiovascular disease, consequences that are especially well documented with regard to soft drinks (carbonated or not). For example, studies involving 88,000 nurses and 42,883 American healthcare professionals have shown that the daily consumption of two servings of soft drinks was associated with a 35% increase in the risk of coronary heart disease. When the amount of added sugar consumed totalled 25% of daily calorie intake, the risk of cardiovascular disease actually tripled. Various factors seem to contribute to the harmful effect of simple sugars: an increase in blood pressure and

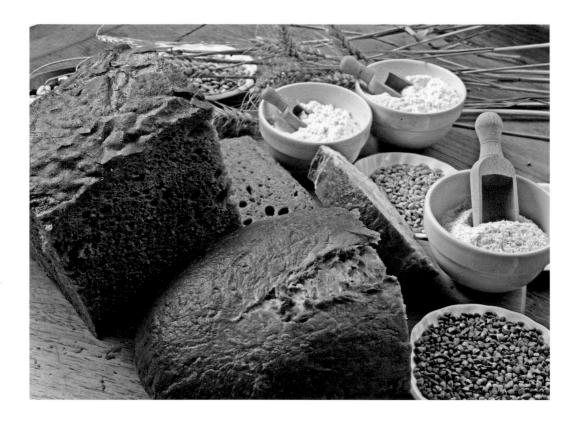

triglyceride levels, a decrease in HDL cholesterol and an increase in LDL cholesterol (more specifically small, very dense LDL that is more harmful for the arteries), increased inflammation, and oxidative stress. Several studies have also shown an increase in numerous inflammation markers that contribute directly to atherosclerosis development. The consumption of added sugars, especially fructose, encourages fat to form in the liver (non-alcoholic hepatic steatosis) and reduces the activity of the lipoprotein lipase in fat cells (adipocytes), reducing the excretion of triglycerides and contributing to abdominal obesity. Fructose also increases the production of uric acid, with the result that less nitric oxide, a powerful vasodilator, is formed. This sugar also stimulates the activity of the sympathetic nervous system and causes sodium retention, contributing to high blood pressure.

According to the World Health Organization, added sugars should not exceed 10% of our daily calorie intake. For an average adult who consumes 2,000 calories a day, this represents 200 calories, the amount in 50 grams or 12 teaspoons of sugar and the equivalent of a single can of pop. The only realistic way to reduce added sugar intake is to limit consumption of processed food products, especially those marketed by the junk food industry, and to completely eliminate soft drinks.

It's also important to note that artificial sweeteners, like aspartame or sucralose (Splenda), do not seem to be acceptable alternative solutions to added sugars. Many studies have clearly established that people who consume foods containing

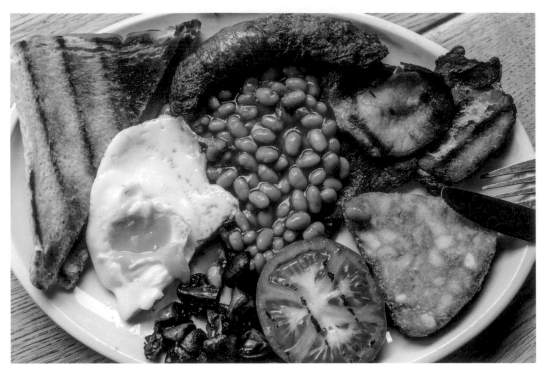

↗ Harmful fats.

these artificial sugars — diet soft drinks, for example — have the same risk of obesity, type 2 diabetes, cardiovascular disease, and metabolic syndrome as those who consume foods containing real sugar. The mechanisms in question remain poorly understood, but it's possible that the brain may be disoriented by the presence of a sweet, calorie-free substance and tries to compensate for this lack by stimulating the appetite. A recent study also suggests that sweeteners trigger changes in the intestinal microbiome, causing glucose intolerance and disruption of the metabolism. So, far from decreasing the damage caused by added sugars, sweeteners may, on the contrary, aggravate these problems.

Another way to reduce the harmful impact of simple sugars on cardiovascular health is to eat whole-grain products whenever possible. In contrast to refined flours that only contain sugar in the form of starch, whole grains also contain the seed coat (the bran) and the embryo (the germ) of the grain; this increases fibre and nutrient intake, while making the sugar in the starch harder to absorb (Figure 27).

As a result, the sugar is released much more slowly, keeping blood sugar at a level high enough to ensure cell function, without, however, reaching levels that are too high and toxic for the body. Fibre slows down gastric emptying, increasing the feeling of fullness and preventing the ingestion of too many calories. It's also fermented in the colon to produce, among other things, short-chain fatty acids with anti-cholesterol and anti-inflammatory properties. The list of benefits associated with consuming dietary fibre is long, and there is no doubt that

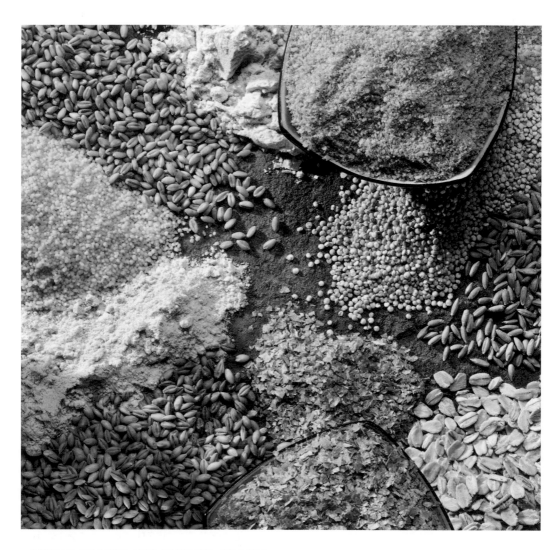

WHOLE GRAINS AND REFINED GRAINS

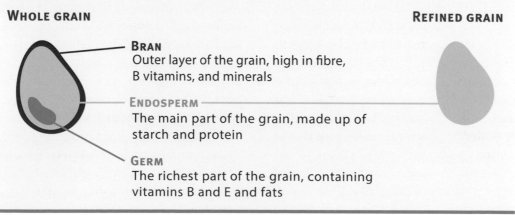

WHOLE GRAIN

REFINED GRAIN

BRAN
Outer layer of the grain, high in fibre, B vitamins, and minerals

ENDOSPERM
The main part of the grain, made up of starch and protein

GERM
The richest part of the grain, containing vitamins B and E and fats

FIGURE 27

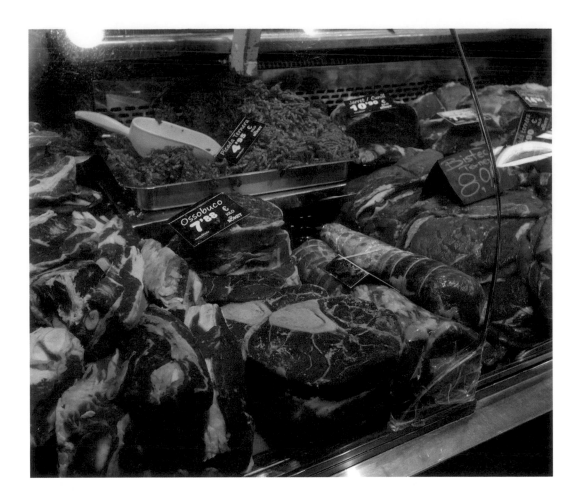

these molecules play a key role in the protective effect of plants on cardiovascular health.

The positive impact of whole grains is clearly illustrated by the reduction in risk of coronary events and mortality observed in a large number of population studies. For example, several meta-analyses have recently shown that consuming roughly 50 g of whole grains per day was associated with a 22% to 30% reduction in mortality from cardiovascular disease, a 14% to 18% reduction in mortality related to cancer, and a 19% to 22% reduction in total mortality.

This protective effect is mainly observed with the fibre in fruits and grains. It's also important to replace refined grain products (bread, rice, white pasta) with their whole-grain equivalents as much as possible. The preventive potential of whole grains remains largely unexploited, as less than 5% of the population eats the three recommended daily servings.

DIVERSITY OF PROTEIN SOURCES

Another consequence of the small amount of plants in our diet is that most of our food proteins come from animal sources, like meat, dairy products, and eggs. Many studies indicate that high consumption of protein from animal sources is associated with a considerable increase in the risk of premature death, a negative impact especially noted for red meat and processed meats. For example, a major study of 121,342 people showed that eating one daily serving of red meat (one hundred grams) and processed meat (fifty grams) increased by 18% and 21%, respectively, the risk of dying from cardiovascular disease. This increase seems to be limited to red meat, as the regular consumption of poultry or fish is instead associated with a decrease in mortality. In several studies, an increased risk of cardiovascular diseases or premature death is especially noted among processed meat consumers. A synthesis of twenty-five studies on 1,218,380 people indicates that, for each serving of fifty grams of processed meat eaten, the risk of coronary disease climbs by 42%, but not for unprocessed red meat. A negative impact of processed meats on blood pressure and the risk of heart failure has also been observed, illustrating just how bad these products are for cardiovascular health. In addition, a study has recently shown that simply replacing processed meats with plant foods lowers the risk of premature death by 34%. As for unprocessed red meat, caution is still advised, since studies have shown that its consumption is associated with weight gain, as well as with an increase in fasting blood sugar and insulin levels, two major risk factors for type 2 diabetes and cardiovascular diseases.

There are really no downsides to diversifying our protein sources and reducing our red meat consumption by replacing it with plant protein sources, such as legumes, nuts, grains, and vegetables. In a large study of eighty-four thousand nurses over more than twenty-six years, Dr. Walter Willett and his colleagues at Harvard University noted that replacing a serving of red meat once a week with a serving of nuts caused a drop of 30% in the risk of a coronary event.

The impact on heart health of the two other major sources of animal protein, dairy products, and eggs, seems more neutral. Drinking milk (two hundred millilitres per day) does not seem to influence the risk of coronary events, stroke, or premature death, despite its high saturated fat content. Some studies suggest that *fermented* dairy products, like yogourt and cheese, might have positive effects on maintaining a healthy body weight, while others claim that these products might even be associated with a lower diabetes risk.

The moderate consumption of low-fat dairy products, especially fermented ones, thus seems to have a neutral and perhaps even positive impact on cardiovascular health. This topic remains a subject of debate, however, since one of these studies, although very well done by a serious author, was partially subsidized by a big yogourt producer. Furthermore, the author is a member of the scientific consultative committee of Global Dairy Platform, a body whose mission is to promote dairy products in the United States.

As for eggs, many studies have shown that their moderate consumption (fewer than seven eggs a week) has no noticeable impact on the risk of heart attack or stroke in the general population, nor in people carrying a genetic variation predisposing them to having a higher LDL cholesterol level (ApoE4). The unlimited consumption of eggs is nonetheless discouraged by a number of experts, like Dr. Jean Davignon of the Montreal Clinical

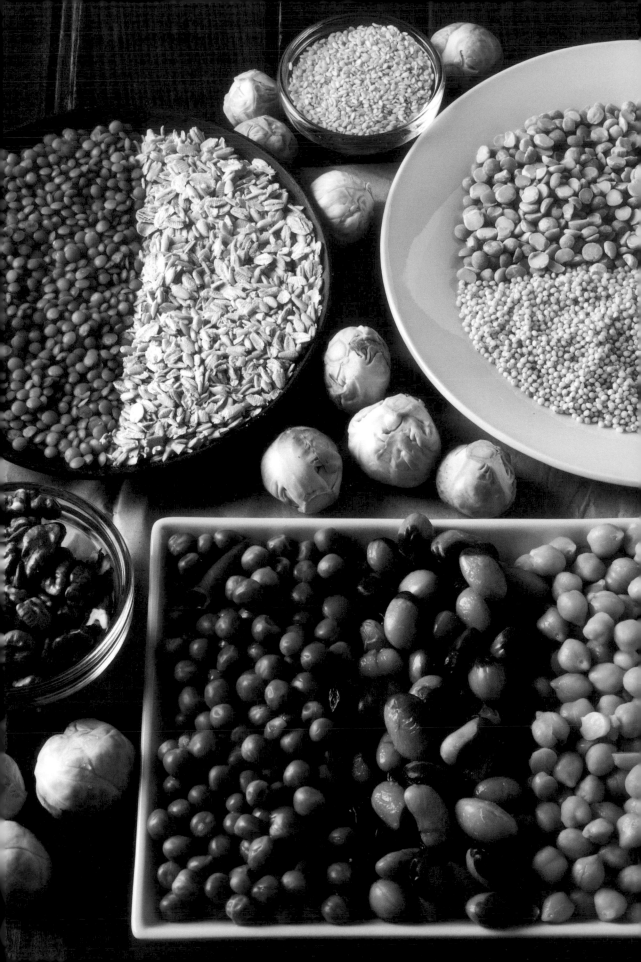

The Intestinal Microbiome: The Billions of Bacteria That Look After Us

The hundreds of billions of bacteria living in our intestine are indispensable partners in maintaining our health. This impressive bacterial community, called the "intestinal microbiome," plays absolutely essential roles in digestion, metabolism, immunity, and even proper brain function. In fact, the microbiome is increasingly considered to be an actual organ, one that must work optimally to keep us in good health.

With respect to cardiovascular diseases, the importance of these bacteria stems from their ability to metabolize certain molecules (phosphatidylcholine, choline, and carnitine) found in animal foods, like meat and eggs. This metabolism generates trimethylamine (TMA), a metabolic "waste" that is transported to the liver, where it's turned into trimethylamine-N-oxide (TMAO), a highly inflammatory molecule. A number of studies indicate that a large amount of TMAO in the blood is associated with the accelerated development of atherosclerotic plaques and an increased risk for cardiovascular disease. One recent study has also shown that the production of TMAO by the intestinal microbiome increased the reactivity of blood platelets and the potential to form blood clots. It's therefore no accident that vegetarians are less likely to develop cardiovascular diseases than carnivores: since they avoid meat, or eat very little, their intestinal bacteria do not generate TMAO, which protects the cardiovascular system.

It's interesting to note that it would also be possible to block the formation of TMAO by acting directly on the metabolism of the bacteria. Indeed, 3,3-dimethyl-1-butanol (DMB), a molecule with a structure analogous to choline, slows down the production of TMAO by various strains of intestinal bacteria and prevents the formation of atherosclerotic plaques in animal models. This natural substance is found in some foods, like red wine and olive oil, two pillars of the Mediterranean diet that have frequently been associated with a significant reduction in heart disease risk. The cardiovascular protection offered by the Mediterranean diet may therefore also stem from a reduction in TMAO formation by intestinal bacteria.

Research Institute (Institut de Recherches Cliniques de Montréal [IRCM]), since one of their properties oxidizes LDL cholesterol and makes it more toxic for the artery walls. A recent study also showed that the phosphatidylcholine in eggs is changed by the intestinal microbiome (see the box above) into an inflammatory molecule, trimethylamine-N-oxide (TMAO), which is harmful to the coronary arteries. People with coronary disease or those at highest risk (those with diabetes, for example) would be wise to limit their consumption to a maximum of one or two eggs a week.

DIFFERENT TYPES OF FAT

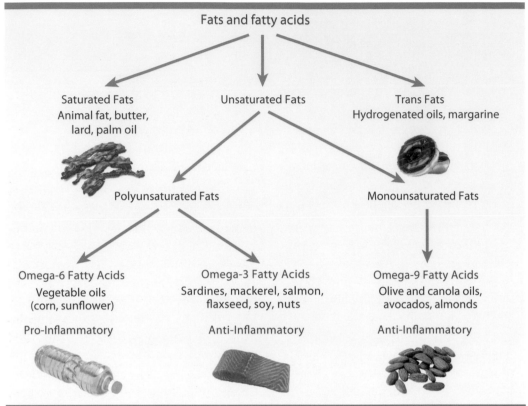

FIGURE 28

CHOOSING YOUR FATS WISELY

Another good reason for replacing animal products with plants is that this substitution also has a positive impact on the kind of fats consumed. Sources of animal proteins (meat, dairy products, eggs) contain saturated fats, whereas fats from plants are mainly unsaturated (Figure 28). These two types of fats have opposite effects on levels of LDL cholesterol: saturated fats are associated with an increase in this cholesterol, while unsaturated fats result instead in a reduction of it.

Studies have shown that simply replacing 5% of calories from saturated fat with sources of unsaturated fat (of the omega-3 type especially) reduces by 10% to 25% the risk of heart attack, as well as cardiovascular mortality. Eating foods high in unsaturated fats, of the omega-3 type from plants (alpha-linolenic acid) or animals (fish), thus becomes very important for cardiovascular health.

Historically, one of the best illustrations of this concept is the dramatic difference in the incidence of cardiovascular disease in some of the world's populations. In 1970, for example, a study showed that inhabitants of the island of Crete, in Greece, who consumed up to 40% of their daily calories in the form of monounsaturated fats (olive oil) and polyunsaturated omega-3 fats were much less affected by these diseases than the Finns, whose main fat intake was of animal origin and therefore saturated (Figure 29). For cardiovascular health, the ideal is therefore to choose unsaturated fat sources like omega-3 vegetable oils, along with nuts, some grains (flax, chia, hemp) and fish, while limiting intake of foods mainly composed of saturated fats, like red meat.

If the superiority of unsaturated fats is so well established, then how can we explain that several studies see no link between the consumption of saturated fats and the risk of cardiovascular disease? You might wonder why you should deprive yourself of butter, cream, and fatty meat if saturated fats have no impact on health. Before jumping to conclusions too quickly, you should know that in numerous studies done in the 1970s and 1980s, the decrease in saturated fat intake was accompanied by a corresponding increase in carbohydrate consumption, mainly in the form of simple sugars, or by higher intake of polyunsaturated omega-6 fats (in fact, saturated fats were replaced by sugars or by lower quality fats). As was mentioned earlier, simple sugars are very damaging for cardiovascular health, not only because they raise triglyceride levels and lower HDL cholesterol, but also owing to their negative impact on increased body weight, high blood sugar levels, insulin resistance (see the box on page 69), and inflammation. In this context, it's normal not to see any advantage to reducing saturated fat consumption; the benefits of this

reduction are quite simply counteracted by the negative impact associated with an increased intake of simple sugars or lower quality fats.

It is not therefore the total amount of fats that matters, but rather the kind of fat consumed. In addition, no study examining the effects of a low-fat diet (in which *all* kinds of fat are reduced) has been able to observe a reduction in the incidence of cardiovascular disease. The best way to maintain an intake of good fats is to choose foods that are good sources of unsaturated fats, while limiting those high in saturated fats. In practical terms, this quite simply means eating more plants (vegetables, legumes, nuts, seeds) and fish, and less red meat, processed meat, and fried foods. Products bearing the words "low-fat" or "0% fat" are not a solution, however, since they were invented by the food industry to profit from the anti-fat fad of the 1980s. They usually contain large amounts of added sugars to make up for the loss of flavour due to the removal of fat and as a result contribute nothing useful in terms of preventing cardiovascular disease. Trans fats must also be completely eliminated (hydrogenated vegetable oil, industrial fat, etc.); these are fats found, for example, in industrially produced croissants, muffins, and cookies, and it has now been clearly established that artificial fats dramatically increase the risk of cardiovascular disease.

In short, the best way to eat well is to adopt a *holistic* view of your diet, without dwelling too much on the individual components of daily foods. Unless you are a nutrition specialist and note systematically all the foods you eat, it's practically impossible to determine precisely the amount of

CHOOSING YOUR FATS WISELY TO PREVENT CARDIOVASCULAR DISEASE

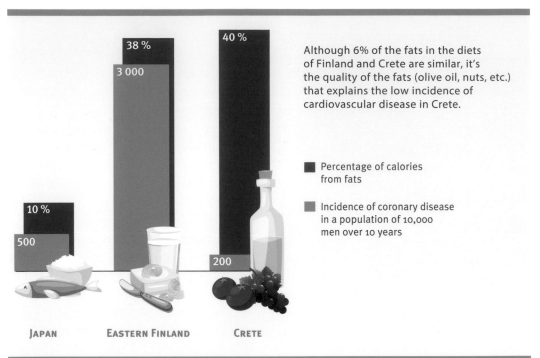

Although 6% of the fats in the diets of Finland and Crete are similar, it's the quality of the fats (olive oil, nuts, etc.) that explains the low incidence of cardiovascular disease in Crete.

■ Percentage of calories from fats

■ Incidence of coronary disease in a population of 10,000 men over 10 years

FIGURE 29   Source: Adapted Stampfer and Willett, 2006

saturated and unsaturated fat or simple sugars consumed every day (all the more so since the numbers on nutrition labels are often imprecise). It's much easier to eat whole foods, mainly plants, limit animal products, and eliminate industrially produced foods as much as possible. For many people, men in particular, meat holds an extremely important place in the diet, and the very idea of eating less of it is immediately viewed as an unacceptable compromise. But a reduction in meat intake, however slight, is associated with health benefits, if this decrease is compensated for by an increase in plant intake. The best example of the benefits of increased plant consumption is without doubt the Mediterranean diet.

Fat and Sugar

In the 1980s, all experts recommended adopting a low-fat diet to reduce blood cholesterol levels and lower the risk of coronary disease. We now know that this anti-fat crusade was a serious mistake: not only did we not make a distinction between good and bad fats, but specialists had also not evaluated the harmful repercussions that could result from replacing fats with other foods, notably those containing added sugars. Consuming too many simple sugars directly contributes to the development of atherosclerosis and promotes weight gain, another risk factor for cardiovascular disease. Some scientists, however, including Dr. Gerald Reaven, had shown in the early 1980s that too many carbohydrates increased the risk for the onset of metabolic syndrome, characterized by insulin resistance, high triglyceride levels, a decrease in HDL cholesterol, an increase in dense LDL (an especially harmful form of LDL), and high blood pressure. But at the time, very few people saw added sugars as harmful substances. The recommendation to reduce fat thus became the norm, supported by an avalanche of industrial food products bearing the words "low-fat" or "0% fat" but containing sometimes astronomical amounts of added sugars.

As Dr. Walter Willett commented later, "By decreasing fats indiscriminately, we have caused an increase in sugar consumption, and this is likely the cause of the obesity epidemic we see today in the United States and elsewhere in the world." Indeed, if we look more specifically at the United States, where data are much more available, we see that there has been, in the last twenty-five years, an increase in calories consumed (about 400 additional calories), an 8% decrease in fats, and a roughly 10% increase in added sugars.

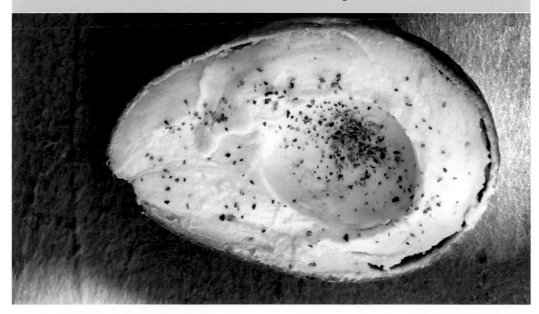

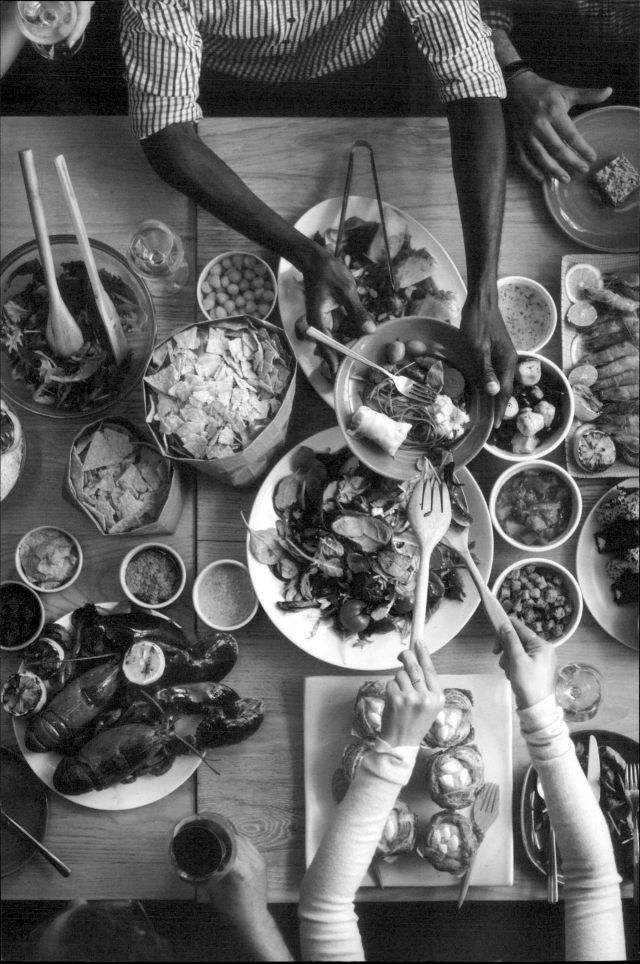

CHAPTER 5

Diet: Effects on Human and Planetary Health

In 2010, the Mediterranean diet was registered by UNESCO on the intangible cultural heritage list as "a set of skills, knowledge, rituals, symbols and traditions concerning crops, harvesting, fishing, animal husbandry, conservation, processing, cooking, and particularly the sharing and consumption of food." This recognition by UNESCO attests to the deep cultural roots at the heart of this diet, but also to its extraordinary impact on health: a vast number of studies have clearly shown that the Mediterranean diet is associated with a major reduction in all chronic diseases, including cardiovascular disease, type 2 diabetes, some types of cancer, and cognitive decline (dementia).

Every culture has its own culinary traditions and there are as many versions of the Mediterranean diet as there are countries in that part of the world. Nonetheless, this type of diet does feature a number of key principles (Figure 30).

Overall, this is a diet high in fruits and vegetables, and in monounsaturated and polyunsaturated omega-3 fats, in which the complex sugars in fibre and grains are the main sources of carbohydrates, and protein comes mostly from legumes, nuts, poultry, and fish, rather than from red meat.

BENEFITS FOR THE HEART

The positive impact of the Mediterranean diet on the prevention of cardiovascular disease was initially suggested by studies comparing the incidence of these diseases in Mediterranean countries with their incidence elsewhere in the world. For example, at the time of these studies, the inhabitants of the Greek islands of Crete and Corfu were largely unaffected by angina, heart attack, and coronary disease

MAIN FOODS IN THE MEDITERRANEAN DIET

Foods Consumed in Large Amounts	Foods Consumed in Moderation	Foods Consumed Occasionally
Monounsaturated fats (olive oil)	Alcohol (red wine)	Red meat and processed meats
Fruits	Fermented or unfermented dairy products	Sweets
Vegetables		
Legumes		
Whole grain products		
Polyunsaturated omega-3 fats (plants or fish)		
Fish		

FIGURE 30

in general. The incidence of these conditions was much lower than in countries where the dietary traditions are mainly based on animal foods, like Finland.

Conducted in the 1990s by French cardiologist Michel de Lorgeril, the Lyon Heart Study is one of the best examples of the great potential shown by the Mediterranean diet for maintaining cardiovascular health. This study aimed to verify the effectiveness of this type of diet in preventing recurrence in people who had suffered a heart attack. The patients were randomly divided into two groups: one group was put on a limited-fat diet, traditionally recommended for cardiac patients, and one group adopted a Mediterranean diet. The results obtained were absolutely astonishing (Figure 31): after four years, among patients who had adopted the Mediterranean diet, the incidence of non-fatal attacks had been reduced by 70% and mortality due to

cardiovascular disease had decreased by 71%, rates twice as high as those obtained with anti-cholesterol medications (see Chapter 9). This study completely revolutionized the nutritional approach taken in cardiology. As a result of many other positive studies, the Mediterranean diet is now recommended by all preventive cardiology experts, both in North America and in Europe.

Not only is the Mediterranean diet beneficial for patients with a coronary disease, it's also effective in primary prevention — in other words, for people who have no cardiovascular disease whatsoever. The PREDIMED Study (Prevención con Dieta Mediterránea) showed that the incidence of cardiovascular disease (heart attack, stroke) decreased by roughly 30% in people eating a Mediterranean diet high in extra-virgin olive oil or in nuts, compared with the control group, who were on a low-fat diet (Figure 32).

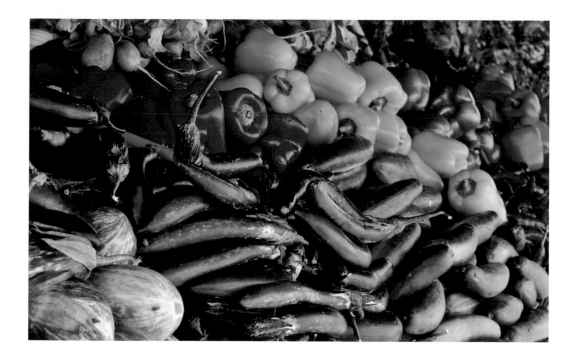

There is therefore no doubt that a Mediterranean-type diet, with its very moderate consumption of meat (about one meal a week), has extremely positive effects on cardiovascular health, both in the general population and in people who have already had a cardiac event.

According to our experience in the last twenty years at the Montreal Heart Institute's EPIC Centre, most people easily adapt to this diet and actually tend to retain their new dietary habits in the long term because they provide such a feeling of well-being.

A PLANT-BASED DIET: REVERSING CORONARY DISEASE

Many studies have shown that people who adopt a mainly plant-based diet are usually in better health and less likely to have cardiovascular disease. Mortality

COMPARISON OF SURVIVAL RATES IN CORONARY PATIENTS ON A LOW-FAT CONTROL DIET OR A MEDITERRANEAN DIET

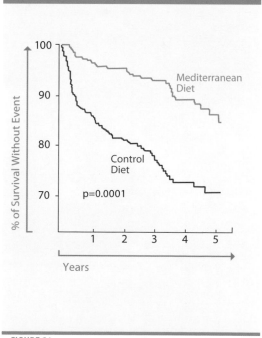

FIGURE 31   Source: De Lorgeril et al., 1999

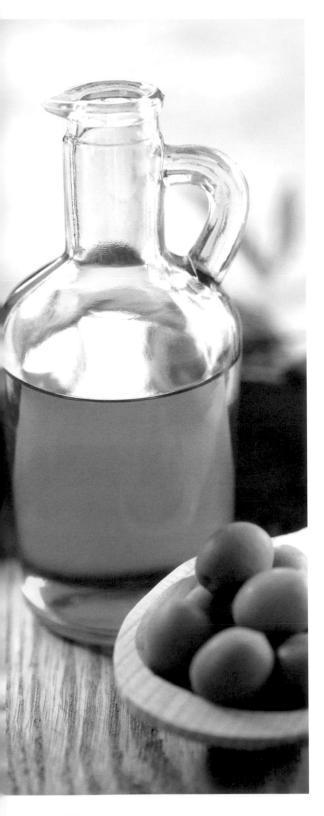

related to coronary diseases is 20% to 30% lower in vegetarians, compared with non-vegetarians; this is especially noticeable in those who have not eaten animal products for at least five years.

For most people, a Mediterranean diet includes sufficient plant intake for them to benefit from this protection. Note that most studies do not indicate that a strictly vegetarian or vegan diet is superior to the Mediterranean diet for preventing cardiovascular disease. For example, an important characteristic of this diet is the regular consumption of fish, and studies confirm that pesco-vegetarians (who eat fish but not meat from "land" animals) have the same low risk of premature death as vegans, who do not eat any animal products, including fish. It should also be noted that strict vegetarianism is very rare in Japan, but that the Japanese, big fish eaters, still have the lowest incidence of cardiovascular disease in the world.

The situation is somewhat different, however, for people with serious coronary disease and who, as a result, are much more likely to die prematurely. Several studies indicate that, for these patients, adopting a strict vegetarian diet without meat or dairy products can halt the progression of atherosclerosis and can even, in some cases, cause the coronary disease to *regress*. The first documented example of this was the case of Dr. Nathan Pritikin, who, at age forty-two, was given a diagnosis of severe coronary disease. Inspired by the low incidence of cardiovascular disease in mainly vegetarian populations, he devised a diet very low in fat and mainly based on a high intake of complex carbohydrates from fruits, vegetables, legumes, and whole grains, combined with frequent but moderate aerobic

PROTECTIVE EFFECT OF THE MEDITERRANEAN DIET

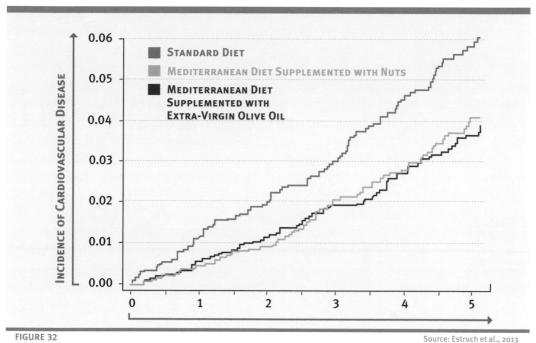

FIGURE 32   Source: Estruch et al., 2013

STENOSIS REGRESSION WITH THE ORNISH PROGRAM

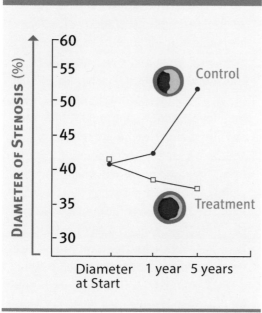

FIGURE 33   Source: Ornish et al., 1998

physical activity. When Dr. Pritikin died of the effects of lymphoma at age 69, pathologists observed that his coronary arteries had only a few small atherosclerosis plaques, a highly remarkable finding in someone of his age who, furthermore, had been diagnosed with serious coronary problems earlier in his life.

Thanks to the cardiac rehabilitation program developed by California doctor Dean Ornish, we now have better documentation of this phenomenon. This program is based on a strict vegetarian diet, high in complex carbohydrates and low in fats, combined with moderate exercise and the application of stress management techniques. Dr. Ornish prescribed this program to patients whose coronary arteries contained large blockages. In addition, they suffered from angina and had abnormal results on stress ECGs, and myocardial perfusion imaging (PET scan) showed a lack of blood in the myocardium (ischemia). A famous study published in 1990 (in *The Lancet*) and in 1998 (in *JAMA*) presented results obtained after one to five years of this treatment, respectively. For this study, Dr. Ornish separated his patients randomly into two distinct groups: one group was subjected to an intensive program, while the other received treatments given according to the standard in cardiology of the time. The results were absolutely amazing: patients following the Ornish method saw their symptoms improve very quickly (in two or three weeks). After one year, a considerable decrease in plaques and a clear improvement in perfusion of the myocardium could be seen. The improvement was even more pronounced after five years. Among patients in the control group, who received the usual treatments, coronary lesions worsened. For example, the severity of the stenosis (blockages) in the vessels of the patients in the control group increased by 11% in the five years following the beginning of the study, whereas it decreased by 3% in those who followed the Ornish method (Figure 33) and by as much as 7% in those who adhered the most strictly to Dr. Ornish's instructions. These reductions may seem modest, but remember that a slight modification in the diameter of an artery causes a large variation in flow, since resistance to blood flow varies exponentially as a function of

A Clinical Example of Coronary Disease Regression

The first patient I put on this program had, at the age of 52, a major blockage (about 80%) in the anterior interventricular artery (the main coronary artery) and experienced stress angina after just five minutes on the treadmill. His cardiologist recommended (correctly) that he have an angioplasty (dilation). By personal choice, this patient wanted a more "conservative" treatment, and was willing only to take medications. His family doctor therefore sent him to me for a second opinion. I explained to him that, if he wanted to avoid a coronary angioplasty, the only option for him would be a very intensive program of lifestyle changes, like the Ornish method, given the severity of his disease. He accepted and adopted a strict vegetarian diet, began doing regular exercise, and undertook a stress management program based on meditation. His situation rapidly improved, to the point where I was able to gradually decrease his medication for angina in a few months. After one year, his electrocardiogram still showed exertional ischemia (lack of blood in the myocardium), but at a very high level (9 METS, or almost twice his capacity before beginning the program), and he no longer had any angina symptoms. I followed up on him annually for ten years or so, before finally "discharging" him. This first case confirmed for me that Dr. Ornish's approach could be adopted by a very motivated person and, since the mid-1990s, I have recommended this "intensive" treatment to patients highly motivated to change their lifestyle habits.

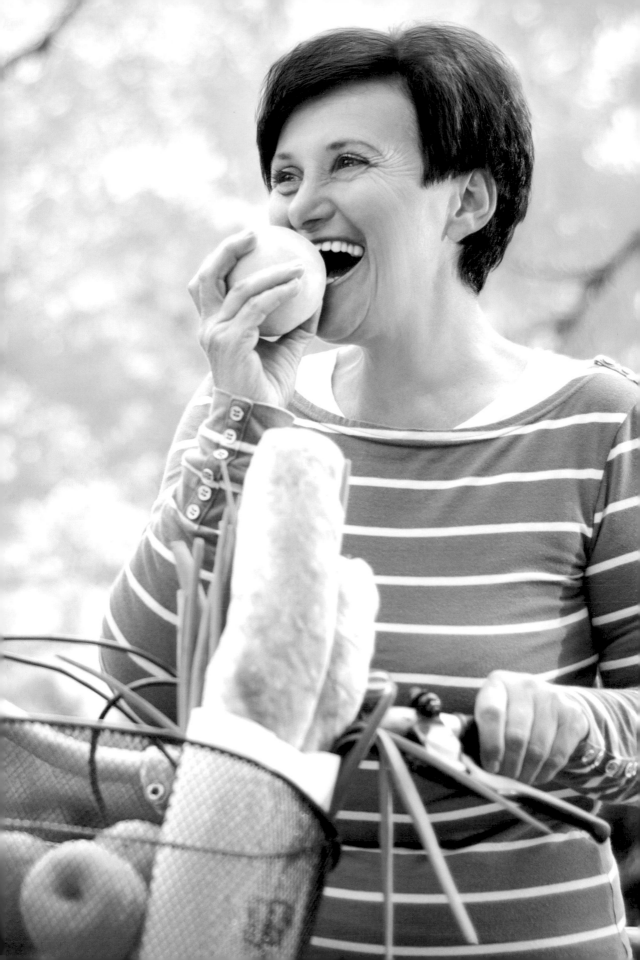

The Ornish Program

I suggest you consult Dr. Ornish's website (www.ornish.com) and watch his lectures on YouTube.

the artery's diameter. As a result, reductions in blockages because of the adoption of the Ornish program led to a notable improvement in myocardial perfusion and the quasi-disappearance of angina symptoms in these patients. In other words, the progression of the coronary disease was not only halted but even reversed in many cases.

Since the publication of these results, the Ornish method has been applied in a great many North American centres with much success. I myself have followed many patients with documented coronary disease who were motivated to follow this rather strict program, and I've witnessed a remarkable evolution. Their symptoms have lessened quickly in a few weeks, to the point where it has been possible to gradually reduce their medication. In most cases, I have never had to operate or dilate the coronaries of patients following the Ornish method, even those whose plaques were numerous and severe.

Another doctor, Dr. Caldwell Esselstyn of the Cleveland Clinic — one of the best cardiology centres in the world — suggests a diet similar to Dr. Ornish's, but does not require his patients to exercise regularly, nor to follow a stress-reduction program. The results obtained are equally excellent; a very favourable evolution in patients is seen, with very rare recurrence of heart attack or severe angina, as well as a notable decrease in medications and surgical treatments. The method used by Dr. Esselstyn is less scientifically rigorous than that of Dr. Ornish (the effects of his diet are not compared with those of a control group, since he believes that a strict vegan diet, very low in fat, is so effective that it would not, according to him, be ethical to treat coronary patients any other way), but it's undeniable that adopting his vegan diet has a very positive impact on the health of his patients. As an example, Figure 34 shows the coronary angiography of a man with severe stenosis of the right coronary artery and indicates that the blockage has definitely shrunk thirty-two months after the adoption of a strict vegan diet.

One of Dr. Ornish's most famous patients is former U.S. president Bill Clinton. After having undergone a quadruple coronary artery bypass in 2004 owing to major blockages in several vessels, Clinton's bypasses rapidly became blocked and had to be dilated

CLINICAL EXAMPLE OF CORONARY DISEASE REGRESSION

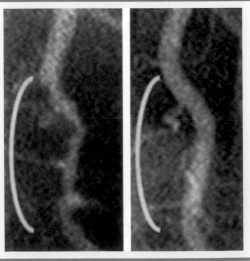

FIGURE 34　　　　　Source: Esselstyn et al., 2014

urgently using coronary angioplasty in 2010. Faced with the dramatic and rapid progression of his heart condition, Clinton got in touch with Dr. Ornish, who recommended his program. In a short time, his medical status improved dramatically, notably because of significant weight loss and the disappearance of his angina symptoms. Today, he claims to be in better shape than ever. For many years now, the Ornish method has not been considered an experimental treatment and therefore is reimbursed in the United States by Medicare, as well as by many private medical insurance companies.

Many North American cardiologists affirm that a diet mainly based on plants, like the one Dr. Ornish suggests, is ideal for cardiovascular health. Dr. K.A. Williams, the outgoing president of the American College of Cardiology, is himself vegan. There is really no controversy about the ability of this kind of diet to counteract atherosclerosis. According to Dr. Williams: "There are two kinds of cardiologists: vegans and those who haven't read the data." Most of my colleagues, however, hesitate to recommend this kind of intensive program, as it's very demanding and it's not, in their view, realistic to ask their patients to become strict vegetarians, exercise three to four times a week, and follow a stress management program. We may, however, ask ourselves which is more radical: to undergo a triple bypass or a coronary angioplasty on two or three vessels or to make major changes to our lifestyle?

My opinion is that patients must be informed of the effectiveness of Dr. Ornish's and Dr. Esselstyn's programs, and then be left to choose. The better informed patients are, the better prepared they are to discuss specific treatment options with their doctor.

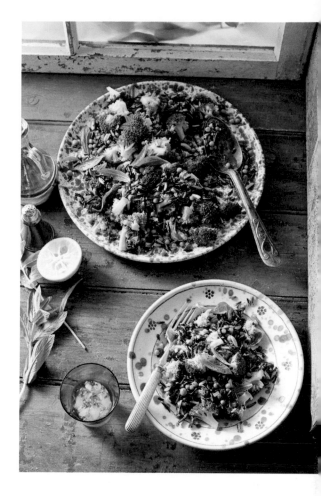

If you already have a documented coronary disease — for example, if you have already had coronary artery bypasses, a coronary angioplasty, or a heart attack, or if you have symptoms of chronic angina — and you are interested in Dr. Ornish's approach, you can discuss it with your doctor.

If you have never had coronary problems, I suggest you adopt the Mediterranean diet, which remains a logical choice for most people. However, if you have several coronary risk factors or if some of your close relatives have had a coronary event at a relatively young age (under sixty-five), I believe you should seriously consider a vegetarian diet. I actually often offer this

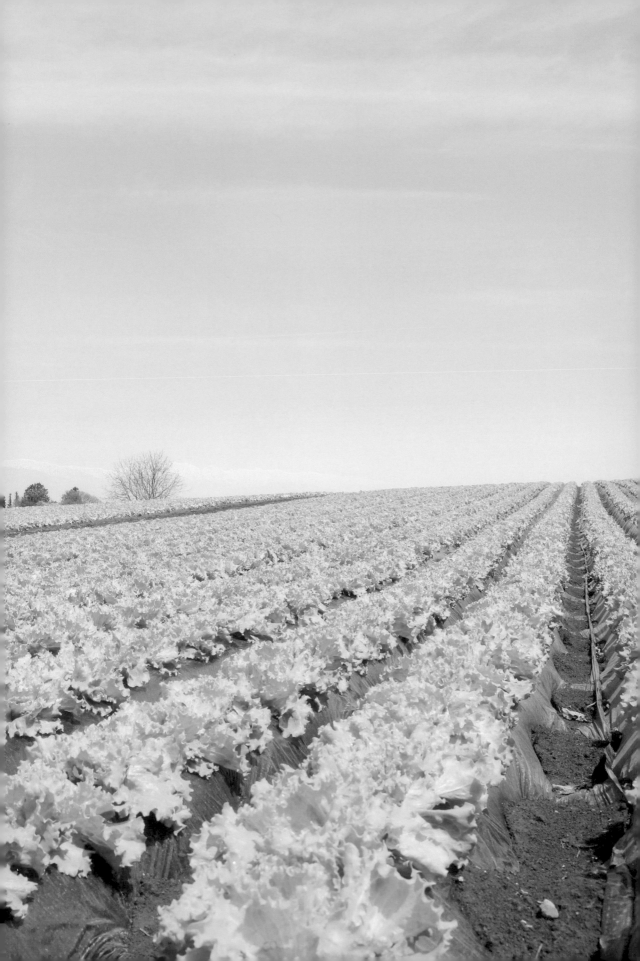

advice to people in their thirties and forties who consult me for a preventive evaluation and who have a lengthy history of cardiovascular disease in their family.

In summary, the risk of cardiovascular disease can be greatly reduced by increasing your intake of plant foods while reducing your consumption of animal products. The decision to adopt a vegetarian or vegan diet must be taken seriously: it's not enough just to cut out meat, since just avoiding meat does not mean that you necessarily eat well. A vegetarian who easts mainly starches (fries, pasta, pastries) or processed food products that imitate meat-based products (tofu sausages, etc.) will obviously not have the best diet possible. Remember that the traditional Mediterranean diet is very much centred on plants, both vegetables and leafy greens, and that these foods play a predominant role in the benefits this kind of diet confers. This is why I always advise my patients who plan to become vegetarian or vegan to consult a nutritionist.

GOOD FOR THE HEALTH OF THE PLANET

In 2006, the United Nations Food and Agriculture Organization (FAO) created a shockwave by publishing a very thorough report showing that livestock farming was responsible for more greenhouse gas (GHG) emissions than the entire transportation industry. According to the FAO, the livestock and dairy industry produces 18% of all GHGs — 9% of the CO_2, 37% of the methane (which has a heating effect at least 25% greater than CO_2), and 65% of the nitrous oxide. Furthermore, livestock farming is the main source of water pollution, in both developed and developing countries.

This assessment by the FAO has been confirmed by other organizations, notably the Intergovernmental Panel on Climate Change (IPCC), which estimates that 25% of GHGs are the result of agriculture, livestock farming, and the ensuing deforestation. Livestock farming is the main cause of these emissions, in particular the manure and methane produced

PRODUCTION OF EMISSIONS IN 2050 AS COMPARED WITH 2009

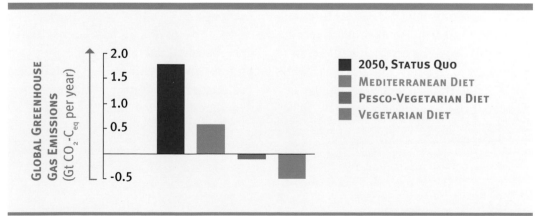

FIGURE 35

Source: Adapted from Tilman & Clark, 2014

by ruminants, which alone are responsible for more than half of GHGs.

The livestock sector also consumes much more protein than it produces: the amount of protein needed to feed livestock is about seventy-seven million tons, whereas the foods produced by the meat of these animals provides just fifty-eight million, a nineteen million ton deficit that could be used to feed human beings. Not to mention that 70% of the total agricultural land surface and 30% of the planet's land mass is used for livestock farming.

In Amazonia, intensive livestock farming is the main cause of deforestation. Since it's predicted that the worldwide consumption of meat will more than double by 2050, the consequences for global warming will be disastrous and will cancel out the positive effects of reducing our oil consumption.

There is no simple solution, as livestock farming is a revenue source for a great many of the world's people, especially in poor countries, where it's estimated to provide the means of subsistence for nearly a billion people. Many experts, on the other hand, recommend at least reducing the projected increase in our meat consumption; this would have a significant impact on global warming and, at the same time, on population health. For example, a recent study published by researchers at Oxford University in England estimates that adopting a Mediterranean diet could reduce the expected rise in GHGs by 2050 by 60%, while pesco-vegetarianism (vegetarianism that includes fish) and vegetarianism could completely cancel out this increase, and even result in emissions below current levels (Figure 35), while considerably reducing mortality related to chronic diseases (cardiovascular disease, diabetes, and various cancers).

Many scientists have published similar studies, and there is no doubt that a decrease in our consumption of animal products could improve both population health and that of the planet. In addition, economically speaking, the reductions in costs for healthcare systems would be as significant, if not more, as the economic benefits related to mitigating climate change.

Given the significant impact of livestock farming on GHGs, it's surprising to see that this problem is rarely discussed at major climate summits. Obviously, this is a complex issue, and pointing fingers at the livestock and dairy production sectors as a whole, as in the case of the petroleum industry, is hard for politicians: it would mean not only taking on a major sector of the economy but also targeting very deeply rooted consumption habits. Suggesting that people eat less meat is much more delicate than asking them to use less oil.

In conclusion, it has been clearly demonstrated that a diet higher in plant proteins and lower in animal proteins has advantages both for the health of individuals and that of the planet.

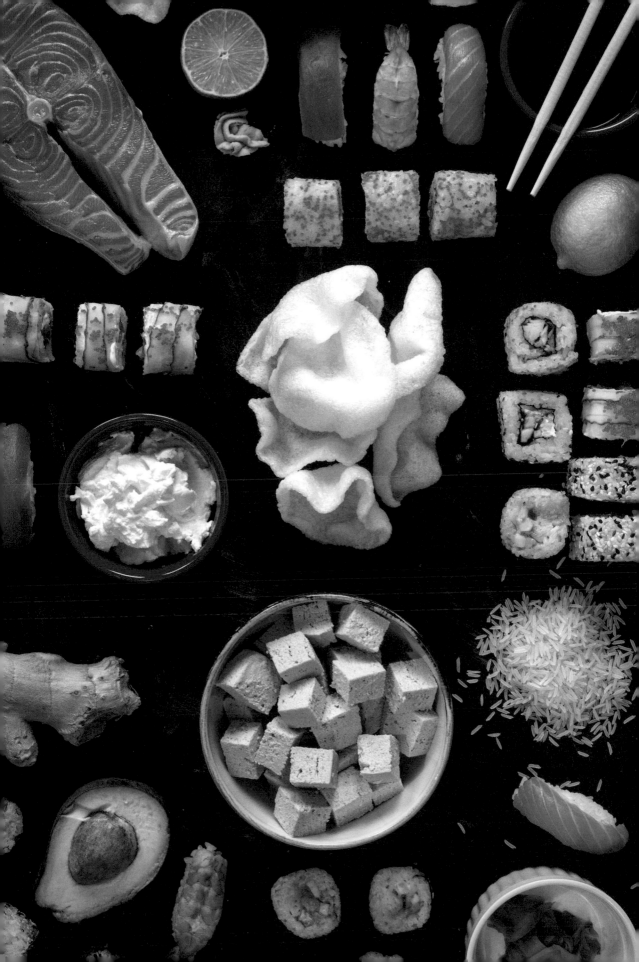

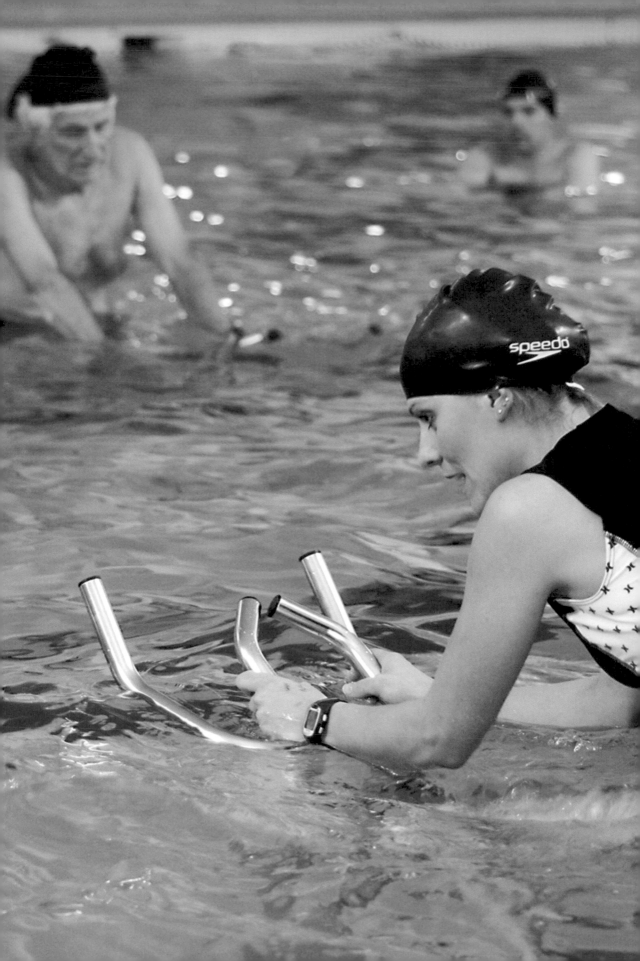

CHAPTER 6

Exercise: The Best Medicine

In human evolution, our physiology adapted to walking and running long distances so we could obtain high-quality food, with enough calories to meet the energy requirements necessary for the functioning and evolution of our brains. Our distant ancestors could actually cover up to twenty kilometres per day (twenty thousand or more steps) to provide for their needs, a physical effort almost four times greater than ours today (Figure 36). This difference is a direct consequence of the profound upheavals in way of life caused by the industrial and technological revolutions of recent decades. Whereas barely a century ago every aspect of daily life required a physical effort, both at work and at home, mechanization and modern technology have made our activities much less physically demanding. One religious community, however, the Amish, rejects this progress and prefers a traditional way of life. Their physical activity is thus similar to that of our ancestors: they walk about fifteen thousand steps a day, whereas an average American adult walks five thousand, or one-third as many. Today, people who drive to work, take the elevator to get to their offices, and spend most of the day in front of a computer do not really use their muscles at all, a situation that can get even worse if they spend their evenings in passive leisure activities in front of a screen (television, tablet, computer). On average, Canadian adults spend nearly ten hours of their waking time in sedentary activities, with no physical activity whatsoever!

This modern sedentary lifestyle has serious consequences for population health: for example, a study done in Australia showed that people who watch television for more than four hours a day experience an 80% increase in their risk of developing cardiovascular disease. An increase in risk for type 2 diabetes and some cancers has also been

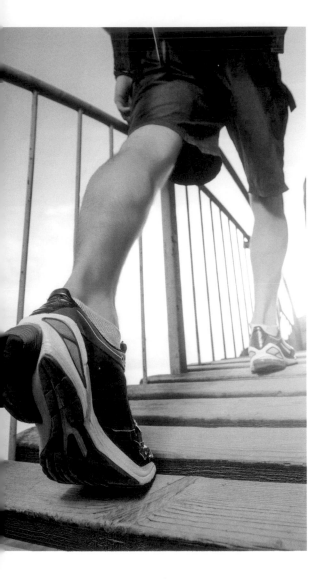

observed in couch potatoes, showing how harmful being inactive for extended periods can be for your health. Unfortunately, according to the Canadian Radio-Television and Telecommunications Commission (CRTC), Canadians spend an average of twenty-eight hours per week in front of the television.

WORKING YOUR HEART OUT

While the importance of physical activity for maintaining good health had already been suggested in ancient times, notably by Hippocrates and Galen, the fathers of medicine, it was not until the middle of the twentieth century that this link could be scientifically established. Credit for this goes to a British doctor, Jeremy Morris, who showed in 1953 that bus drivers in London, seated at the wheel all day, had more cardiovascular events than ticket inspectors, who went from one deck to another to check tickets (Figure 37A). A similar situation was also observed among British civil servants: those who were more physically active, letter carriers, for example, had half as many cardiovascular events as their fellow workers in more sedentary jobs,

IMPACT OF INDUSTRIALIZATION ON NUMBER OF STEPS PER DAY

Population	Year	Average Number of Daily Steps
Paleolithic	20,000 years ago	10,560 to 21,120
Amish	2002	14,196 to 18,425
Americans	2010	4,912 to 5,340

FIGURE 36

Source: Adapted from Booth, 2012

like telephone operators and office clerks (Figure 37B).

Although remarkable, these results were received at the time with great skepticism by the medical community, as doctors did not believe that something as simple as physical activity could influence the risk of coronary disease. Doctors also criticized the methodology Dr. Morris used, stressing that the driver might have this job because he was already less healthy than someone who could walk around and climb the stairs of a double-decker bus all day long. This famous "selection bias" has always been the Achilles heel of epidemiological studies of physical activity: are people who get more physical activity, who have fewer cardiovascular events and who have a longer life expectancy not simply healthier to start with than those who don't? In other words, those who do no physical activity are inactive because they are already ill, and it's therefore normal for them to be more likely to die prematurely than people in better shape.

In the years that followed, many studies were nonetheless able to resolve this problem and clearly establish that regular physical activity is closely associated with a decrease in the incidence of cardiovascular disease. Dr. Ralph Paffenbarger, a famous researcher at Stanford University in California, showed that port employees in the city of San Francisco who were assigned to office work had a coronary mortality rate 80% higher than those who unloaded ships and were as a result much more active. Since these jobs were assigned according to very strict union rules that did not take into account the workers' state of health, these results indicated that it was work related physical activity that was mainly responsible for this difference in risk. A similar situation has been

INCIDENCE OF HEART ATTACK AND PREMATURE MORTALITY

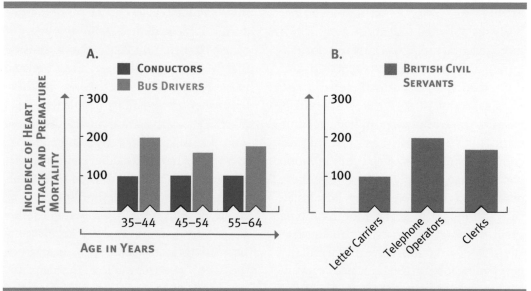

FIGURE 37

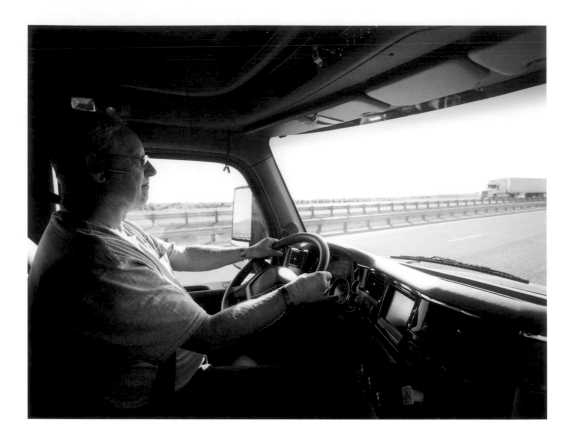

observed in workers on Israeli kibbutzes, the collectivist communities based on joint property ownership. By comparing the physical activity levels of workers on these kibbutzes, it was established that those assigned to more sedentary tasks (accountants, for example), had twice the heart attack risk of those whose work required more intense physical activity (like farmers and cooks). Because the kibbutzniks all had the same standard of living, ate the same food (in a common canteen), and had similar blood cholesterol and triglyceride levels, these observations were able to show how much the simple fact of doing a job requiring greater energy expenditure influences the risk of premature death. Physically demanding jobs thus significantly prevent cardiovascular disease.

In most cases, on the other hand, work requires only very little physical effort, and it's absolutely necessary to compensate for this sedentariness by getting more exercise during our leisure time. A lifestyle study of 16,963 Harvard University alumni showed that the risk of heart attack is directly related to the amount of energy used during these leisure periods: sedentary people were 64% more likely to have a heart attack than those who were much more active. Subsequently, more than a hundred studies confirmed that physical exercise lowered the risk of cardiovascular events, whether heart attack, stroke, or sudden death. Many studies have also clearly demonstrated that regular physical activity is associated with a decrease in the risk of developing at least thirteen different kinds of cancer, type 2 diabetes, and

cognitive decline. The list of the health benefits of exercise is very long (Figure 38) and,
as the saying goes, "If a pill could provide
all the benefits of physical activity, it would
become an instant worldwide success."

MINIMUM EFFORT

Not only are the benefits of physical
activity numerous, the amount of exercise
required to make the most of these benefits is much lower than you might think.
Until quite recently, it was thought that an
energy expenditure of one thousand calories a week was the minimum amount
necessary to decrease the risk of premature
death. This corresponds to sixty minutes
of low-intensity activity, thirty minutes
of medium-intensity activity, or twenty
minutes of high-intensity activity per day,
every day of the week (Figure 39).

However, a very large study done in
Taiwan has overturned this notion. By
examining the physical activity levels of
almost half a million men and women over
eight years, researchers have shown that as
little as fifteen minutes of moderate physical activity per day (walking, for example)
is sufficient to noticeably reduce the total
number of deaths, as well as the mortality
rate associated with cardiovascular disease,
diabetes, and some cancers.

Obviously, the extent of these benefits will be even greater if the duration and
intensity of the physical activity performed
is increased (Figure 40). For example, while
15 minutes of moderate activity like walking
reduces the risk of premature death by 14%,
this risk will be decreased by nearly 20%
if we walk for 30 minutes and reaches a
maximum of about 35% with 90 minutes of

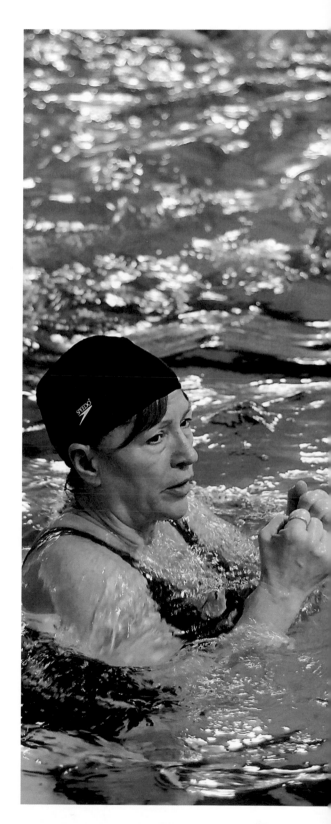

THE MANY BENEFITS OF REGULAR PHYSICAL EXERCISE

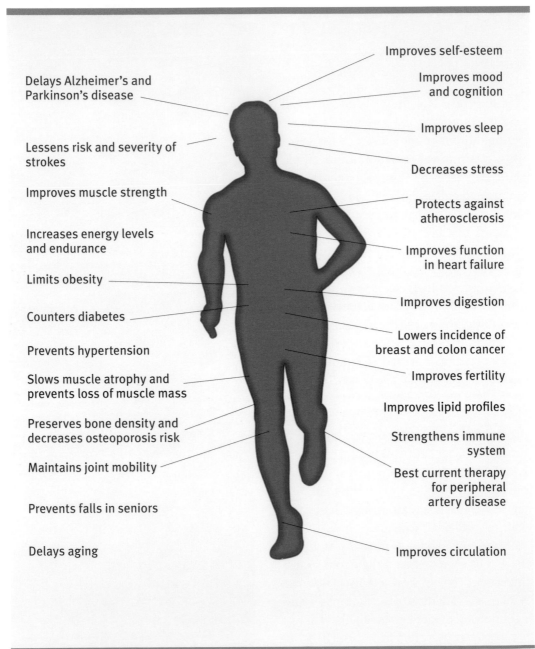

Improves self-esteem

Improves mood and cognition

Delays Alzheimer's and Parkinson's disease

Improves sleep

Lessens risk and severity of strokes

Decreases stress

Improves muscle strength

Protects against atherosclerosis

Increases energy levels and endurance

Improves function in heart failure

Limits obesity

Improves digestion

Counters diabetes

Lowers incidence of breast and colon cancer

Prevents hypertension

Improves fertility

Slows muscle atrophy and prevents loss of muscle mass

Improves lipid profiles

Preserves bone density and decreases osteoporosis risk

Strengthens immune system

Maintains joint mobility

Best current therapy for peripheral artery disease

Prevents falls in seniors

Delays aging

Improves circulation

FIGURE 38

Source: Adapted from Rowe, 2014

walking per day. In practical terms, the message to retain is that the simple fact of performing from 15 to 60 minutes of moderate exercise daily provides major health benefits. And this is true at any age: a study done in Hawaii showed that people 65 and over who walked 3.2 kilometres or more each day had half the premature mortality risk of sedentary people.

These benefits can, however, be achieved much faster through vigorous exercise like running. Running fast for just 5 minutes provides the same benefits as a 15-minute walk, while a 25-minute run equals 105 minutes of walking, making it four times as effective (Figure 40).

In other words, the more vigorous or intense the physical activity, the less time it takes to see benefits in terms of reducing the risk of premature death. Similar results have been obtained in a study done among 55,137 American adults: compared with people who never ran, runners had 45% less risk for cardiovascular disease and their risk of premature death was reduced by 30%, which translates into an additional three years of life expectancy. And here, too, the amount required is much lower than the usual recommendations (75 minutes of vigorous exercise a week). So running less than fifty-one minutes *a week*, or five to ten minutes per day, even at a relatively low speed (less than six kilometres per hour), is enough to considerably reduce early death. Running longer is not associated with a notable increase in this protective effect, an observation confirmed by many studies showing that very intense and vigorous exercises, like those performed by athletes, do not seem to reduce the risk of premature mortality or cardiovascular disease to a greater degree.

You do not, therefore, have to train to the point of exhaustion or spend long hours at

DURATION AND FREQUENCY REQUIRED TO BURN ROUGHLY 1,000 KCAL PER WEEK DEPENDING ON INTENSITY OF PHYSICAL ACTIVITY

Intensity (Category)	Frequency (Number of times per week)	Duration (Minutes)	Kcal/Session
Low	7	60	150
	4	90–120	250
Moderate	7	30	150
	4	45	250
High	7	20	150
	4	30	250

FIGURE 39

the gym lifting weights to enjoy the benefits of physical activity on health. Our society places enormous emphasis on elite sports (the Olympic Games, world championships, extreme sports), which may give the impression that getting exercise is all about spectacular athletic performances or breaking records. This is completely false, as research clearly shows that incorporating just five to fifteen minutes of vigorous exercise or thirty minutes of moderate activity into your daily routine is more than enough to considerably reduce the risk of premature death, enjoy a wide range of health benefits, and noticeably improve quality of life.

The positive impact of physical activity is very well illustrated by the work of James Fries, a Stanford University researcher. For several years, his research team has been monitoring a cohort of occasional, but regular, runners in the Palo Alto area of California and periodically compares their state of health with a group of sedentary people of the same age. The results are truly extraordinary and show that, as they age, especially after 75, physically active people have a much lower level of disability than sedentary people (Figure 41). This study proves that the level of disability of active people is very low, even at 80 years of age and over, while that of sedentary people is quite high, from 75 years of age onward. In fact, the period of disability of active people is usually *eight years shorter*, on average, than that of sedentary people. This is called "compression of morbidity." Thus, rather than trying to prolong life, health interventions should instead aim to compress the period of morbidity at the end of life, so that everyone can live as long as possible in good health before dying.

COMPARISON OF THE BENEFITS OF WALKING AND RUNNING

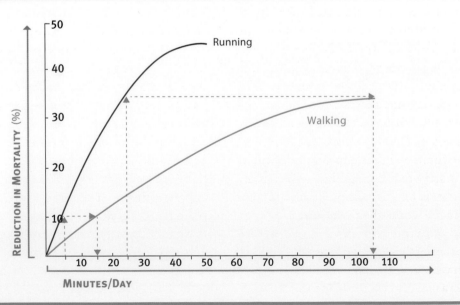

FIGURE 40

Source: Adapted from Wen, 2014

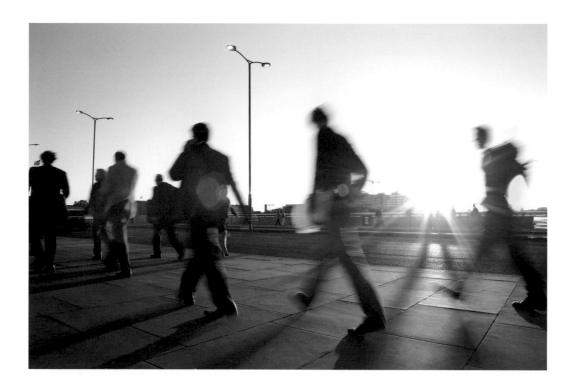

EXTREME EXERCISE

On September 13 in 490 BCE, the Athenians won a major victory fighting the troops of the Persian king Darius I at the battle of Marathon, a city northeast of Athens. According to legend, Phidippides the Greek ran the forty-two kilometres between the two cities to announce the good news to the Athenians, but he just had time to deliver his message (*"Nenikekamen!"* meaning "We have won!") before collapsing and dying. A tragic story that nonetheless served as the inspiration for the most popular endurance test in the world: the marathon.

A growing number of people are attracted by these demanding competitions. Each year more than half a million runners finish a marathon in the United States alone. And this is not to mention the extreme endurance runs that have sprung up in recent decades, like the ultra-marathons of 218 kilometres (in Death Valley in the United States) or 240 kilometres (Marathon des sables in Morocco); the Ironman triathlon (3.8 kilometres of swimming and 180.2 kilometres of cycling, followed by a marathon); or even the ultra-triathlons, like the triple deca-Ironman (an Ironman each day for thirty days)! These performances are quite simply unbelievable, but I always tell my patients who want to train for this type of event that they must do so only if it's their passion and not with the aim of being in better health. As was mentioned earlier, there is absolutely no purpose in training this much just to prevent cardiovascular disease and live longer, since maximum protective effect is reached at levels of physical activity much lower than these extremes.

Of greater concern are studies showing that intensive and prolonged physical

DISABILITY AS A FUNCTION OF AGE IN RUNNERS AND SEDENTARY PEOPLE

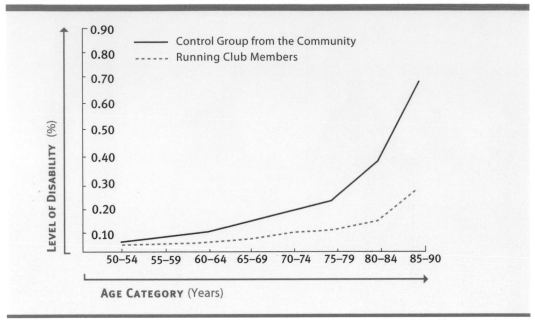

FIGURE 41   Source: Adapted from Wang et al., 2002

activity can cause a number of cardio-vascular complications. It has long been known that the hearts of athletes who train very hard can become different from those of the general population, owing to hypertrophy of the left ventricle and a thickening of the wall of the cardiac muscle. These changes reflect the normal adaptation of the heart to the enormous workload imposed by intensive training, such as that done by elite athletes in dis-ciplines that combine strength and aero-bics (rowing, cross-country skiing, cycling, swimming). At rest, the heart pumps about five litres of blood a minute and this flow can be multiplied by five or even by seven during very high-intensity exercise — reaching twenty-five to thirty-five litres a minute. This dramatic increase in blood flow obviously has repercussions for the cardiac muscle, when a workload like this

is repeatedly imposed. Physiological adap-tation to regular exercise is completely normal and beneficial. However, studies indicate that performing an activity very intensively for more than twenty hours a week over several years can result in arrhythmias, like atrial fibrillation.

This heart rhythm anomaly is usually seen in people over 65 and is characte-rized by very irregular heartbeats, a result of malfunction in the electrical activity in the left atrium (the ventricles contract nor-mally, fortunately). The transmission of the electrical signal becomes so erratic that the atrium does not contract, causing a pooling of blood in the atrium and a high risk of clot formation (thrombus). This clot can at any moment pass through the mitral valve, enter the left ventricle, and from there be ejected into the bloodstream through the aorta (Figure 42).

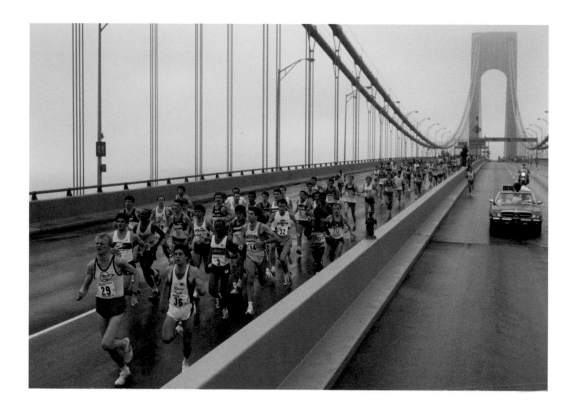

Often, the clot will then travel to the brain and cause a cerebral embolism, with devastating consequences. Atrial fibrillation left untreated by anticoagulants is in fact one of the main causes of strokes.

A relationship between long-term, intensive exercise and arrhythmia like this is suggested by studies showing that the greatest athletes, such as marathoners, cyclists, and professional or high-level cross-country skiers, are the most affected by atrial fibrillation. For example, one study showed that Scandinavian cross-country ski champions who had completed the most races with the best times were four or five times as likely to have episodes of atrial fibrillation. This increased risk does not appear to be limited to elite athletes; it also seems to affect men under 50 who train *very intensively* more than five days a week. How this works has been the subject of numerous studies,

the best known having been done by Dr. Stanley Nattel's team at the Montreal Heart Institute, in which rats were subjected to intensive training on a treadmill one hour per day for sixteen weeks straight, equal to ten years of human training. The results showed that atrial fibrillation appears to be related to a dilation of the atria caused by increased blood flow, as well as by a hyperactivity of the vagus nerve that makes the atrium more likely to contract haphazardly. Conversely, to complicate things somewhat, regular *moderate* physical activity contributes to a decreased risk of atrial fibrillation. Everything thus depends on the "dose" of exercise.

Furthermore, in high performance athletes, other studies have revealed fibrosis in different parts of the right and left ventricles that can lead to dangerous ventricular arrhythmias.

ATRIAL FIBRILLATION IS A COMMON CAUSE OF STROKE

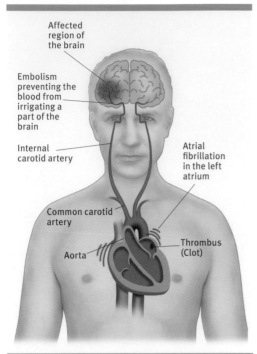

FIGURE 42

Remember that exercise is indispensable for preventing cardiovascular disease and for maintaining overall good health, but that it's better to exercise moderately and not go to extremes so as to avoid problems associated with prolonged periods of very intensive training.

We must be especially wary of the longer-term complications of "extreme" exercise, in particular the increased risk of atrial fibrillation. Even though they are dramatic and always make the headlines, sudden deaths like that of Phidippides are still very rare: between January 2000 and March 2010, there were only 59 sudden deaths among 10.9 million marathon and half-marathon runners, equal to an incidence of 0.5 deaths

per 100,000 participants. A higher mortality rate has been noted in triathlons (1.5 deaths per 100,000 athletes with most of these deaths occurring in the first segment of the event, the swimming portion).

BRIEF BUT INTENSE

For those who enjoy the feeling associated with intense physical activity, one possible option is intermittent high-intensity exercise, also known as "interval training." Initially, this method was developed in the 1930s and 1940s to train (successfully) specific athletes, notably the Swede Gunder Hägg (1918–2004), holder of a dozen world records in athletics. Intermittent high-intensity exercise has been studied scientifically by German cardiologist Herbert Reindell, who noted that alternating short periods of intense effort with periods of low-intensity activity resulted in increased exercise capacity (Figure 43). Interval training has been quickly adopted by high-level athletes, amateur athletes, and, more recently, the general public.

The principle behind this kind of training is very simple. Instead of being done continuously and moderately, for example for 30 or 40 minutes, it's done in a shorter period, say 15 minutes, consisting of short very fast intervals followed by brief rest periods. At the MHI's EPIC Centre, we have studied dozens of interval training protocols and the one our members prefer is the following: fifteen seconds of stationary cycling at maximum capacity, followed by fifteen seconds of complete rest, for eight minutes. You thus pedal for a total of four minutes. There is then a short four- or five-minute pause

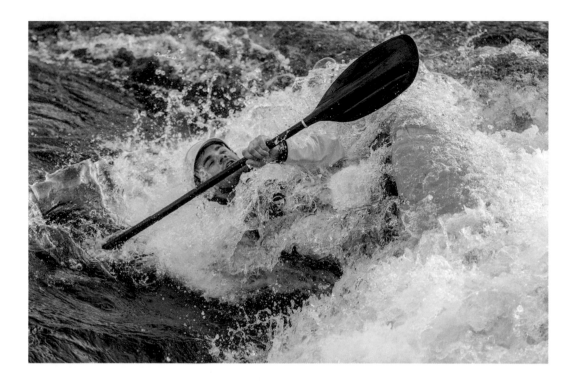

for stretching and relaxation exercises, and then you start all over again for a second eight-minute period. In total, you do sixteen minutes of physical activity, but only eight minutes of actual activity, since you are resting half the time. When aerobic capacity is measured after this kind of training, it's noted that these eight minutes of intense physical activity, split up, are more effective than thirty minutes of continuous moderate activity. Recent studies even suggest that as little as three minutes of intense activity per week, split up into twenty-second blocks, would be enough to increase aerobic capacity!

There is therefore no doubt that interval training is very good for increasing aerobic capacity, but it's obvious that not everyone likes it. Many of my patients, even the very elderly, like this kind of training because "it goes faster" or "it's more fun," while others find on the contrary that it's "too

aggressive" and prefer to stay with "normal" continuous moderate physical activity, like walking. But since the most difficult thing is to maintain the effort over the long term and not to abandon it after only a few months, I advise varying the kind of physical activity you do as much as possible by incorporating interval training into your routine from time to time. Doing different exercises in different ways maximizes the likelihood of continuing to exercise for life. That's what counts.

NOT TO LOSE WEIGHT!

Over the years, physical exercise has usually been considered a way of "burning" extra calories so as to maintain a normal weight. This message is misleading for two main reasons. First of all, it's very simplistic: regular physical activity

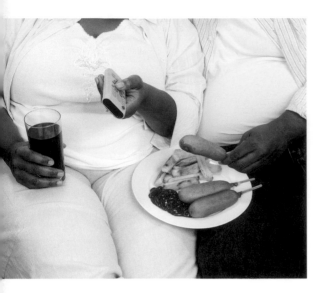

regularly performed a high-intensity physical activity for 20 years gained weight anyway. Obviously, they put on less than people who remained sedentary, but the impact of the exercise remained relatively modest. Scientific data gathered for the past 30 years indicate clearly that people get as much physical activity now as during the last three decades, and that sedentariness cannot explain the phenomenal increase in the number of people who are overweight or obese. It's actually the calories consumed that are the problem, a direct consequence of the massive arrival on the market of calorie-dense foods, found everywhere and often in enormous servings.

offers benefits that go far beyond weight management, including in particular a notable reduction in the risk of cardiovascular disease as well as an increase in longevity and quality of life. The other problem with this message is that it's largely untrue, since it's much more the *amount of energy consumed* that determines the accumulation of excess fat than the level of physical activity. For example, one study has shown that men and women who

Not surprisingly, therefore, the food industry, especially the junk food industry, is the main promoter of exercise as a way of controlling body weight, and it continuously repeats that the obesity epidemic is due to a sedentary lifestyle rather than the increase in number and decrease in quality of calories consumed. All of the big junk food companies, whether

PRINCIPLE OF INTERVAL TRAINING

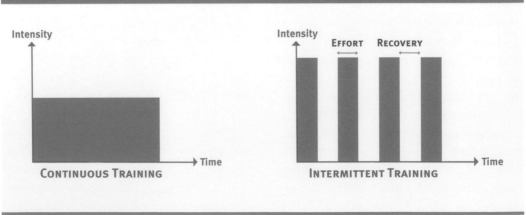

FIGURE 43

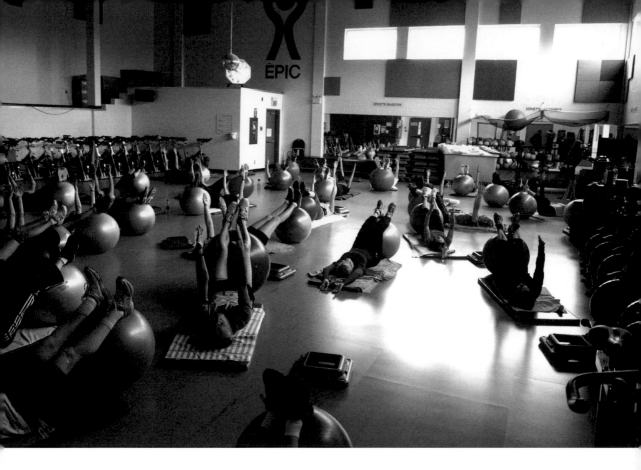

Coca-Cola, Pepsi, Hershey's, or McDonald's, persist in claiming that it's all a question of balance and that the obesity problem is secondary compared with a lack of physical activity. This also explains why these companies sponsor major sports events like the Olympic Games or the World Cup of soccer, to name but two.

I'm not saying that exercise is not important in the fight against obesity. In fact, recent studies indicate that it's associated with a significant decrease in visceral fat (located in the abdomen) and with the amount of fat stored in the liver, two significant risk factors for cardiovascular disease. But as a way of shedding a substantial number of excess kilograms, exercise does not carry much weight (no pun intended), compared with the amount of calories consumed. For example, to burn

100 calories, an adult man weighing 70 kilograms has to walk 1.6 kilometres. If he eats just one piece of sugar pie, containing nearly 400 calories, he will have to walk *about 6.5 kilometres* to burn off these excess calories (depending on your height and weight, this number varies from 5 to 8 kilometres)! Examples like this are easy to find in fast food restaurants. For example, the Blizzard (an ice cream sold by a well-known chain) can contain more than 1,000 calories, easily consumed in less than five minutes. Imagine the enormous amount of exercise it would take to burn them off (you would have to walk 16 kilometres)! It must also be understood that our body has changed during evolution to resist famines and that it is, as a result, extremely efficient at *storing* calories during periods of deprivation.

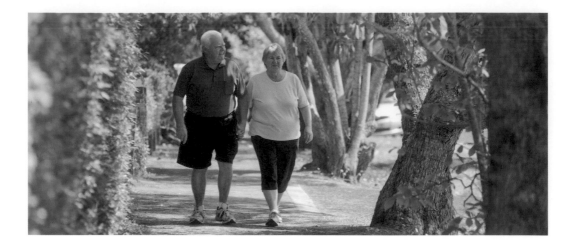

MOTIVATED TO GET MOVING

The most important thing to do to remain motivated is to focus each day on the benefits of physical activity. After a session of moderate exercise, we feel good; the trick is to "sustain" this feeling of well-being, so that we are encouraged to do it again the next day or the day after. Setting long-term objectives is harder, since our psychology is such that a far-off benefit is not the best motivation.

The kind of exercise or where you do it is of little importance. Some years back, it was thought that only aerobic training was good for cardiovascular health, but now we know that strength training is also excellent. A complete training program must include some kind of aerobic activity and a period of strength training, as well as work on balance and flexibility. Kinesiologists are the professionals best trained to advise you on various kinds of exercise. I recommend that everyone meet with one of these specialists at least once to have a physical activity program designed that is aligned with their preferences and respects their limitations. This is a minimal investment that's really worth it.

AIR POLLUTION AND CARDIOVASCULAR DISEASE

Unfortunately, air pollution is a factor that must be considered before starting a physical activity. A great many studies have shown that this kind of pollution, especially when it contains fine and ultrafine particles (transport emissions), is very harmful to the cardiovascular system; the particles easily penetrate the lungs, pass directly into the pulmonary blood vessels, and from there move into all the arteries in the body. There they produce an inflammatory reaction and damage the vascular endothelium, the fine layer of cells that covers the internal wall of the arteries and ensures they function properly. The arteries then dilate less easily and as a result have a greater tendency to contract, impairing normal blood circulation. If this effect is combined with increased blood coagulation (the prothrombotic effect), all the conditions are then in place to cause cardiac events and strokes or exacerbate an existing coronary disease.

Unfortunately, there are few options when the air pollution in your region is high. A notice from the American Heart Association published in 2010 suggests avoiding *intensive exercise* (jogging and other vigorous physical activities) when the air quality index is poor. This recommendation is based on studies showing that, during exposure to high levels of fine particles, their inhalation is 4.5 times greater during physical effort than while resting. Another study reported that, in heavy traffic, cyclists were 4.3 times more exposed to air pollutants than passengers in cars travelling in the same areas. People who already have cardiovascular disease or diabetes and the elderly are especially at risk, but the authors of this notice recommend that everybody reduce the intensity of physical activities and choose indoor training, even though the air inside buildings may also be polluted if there is no effective filtration system. The authors also strongly suggest avoiding intensive exercise during rush hours and near places where the traffic is very heavy.

In Montreal, according to the city's environment service, there were 63 days of poor air quality in 2014 and 64 days in 2015, attributable to fine particles, among other things, including 10 days of smog in the winter. The situation is often worse in winter, since heating with wood comes in second, after vehicle emissions, as a cause of fine particle emissions ($PM_{2.5}$). There are several Internet sites where air quality in every region can be checked daily. These information sites are very useful, as exceptional circumstances can seriously alter air quality: that's what happened on May 22, 2016, when the air quality index (which takes into account fine particles and various gas pollutants) was 106 in Montreal, higher than in Beijing (93), New York (56), Paris (41), and Los Angeles

(26). Luckily, this was an exceptional situation, caused by a specific anticyclone system that kept the polluted air over the city.

To get the maximum benefit from exercise without spending too much time, walking, jogging, or cycling moderately for thirty to forty minutes, three or four times a week is recommended. To determine whether an exercise is moderate, do the "talk test": if you can sustain a conversation during your activity, it's moderate. When you can no longer speak normally, this indicates that the exercise is more intense. This is a little harder, but offers more advantages, both for mind and for health, in less time.

For people who like numbers, we usually say that training is effective when the heart rate reaches between 65% and 90% of its maximum rate. The latter is determined by the following formula: 220 minus the individual's age. However, this is a rough approximation, since maximum heart rate varies considerably from one individual to another. The only way to determine your heart rate precisely is to take a maximal stress test on a bicycle or treadmill, but it's neither realistic nor desirable to subject the entire population to this kind of test before beginning an exercise program. We can instead rely on people's perception of effort. Swedish psychologist Gunnar Borg clearly showed that this perception is even more reliable than heart rate measured by a heart rate monitor to estimate the level of intensity of the effort.

Our brain is a very good judge, as it's able to take into account simultaneously respiratory rate, the feeling of fatigue, and various other physiological parameters (like lactic acid in the muscles, which causes heaviness in the legs

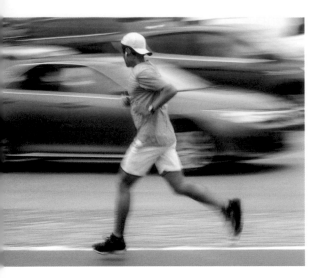

during intense exercise). This is why I often tell my patients that the intensity level reached during the activity must not cause major discomfort. If, however, you like to feel slight discomfort, it should be quite brief, no more than a few minutes. If you are not a high-performance athlete and you constantly train beyond your limits over long periods, exercise sessions will be painful, and you will need several hours to fully recover. Proper training will leave you with a feeling of well-being and invigorate you rather than exhausting you.

GETTING A MOVE ON AFTER A HEART ATTACK

Up to the end of the 1960s, heart attack victims were advised to stay in bed for a month. The intention was to protect the heart, but it was subsequently shown that this forced rest was associated with a major deterioration in cardiac and muscle function, and that a more rapid return to

normal activities was desirable. One of the first to advocate a faster return to physical activity after a heart attack was Dr. Paul Dudley White, an eminent cardiologist at Massachusetts General Hospital in Boston, considered the "father" of American cardiology. When American president Dwight Eisenhower had a heart attack on September 24, 1955, Dr. White advised him to adopt a regular exercise program, a "prescription" that was adopted two decades later by the entire medical community. The wisdom of this approach was confirmed by the famous Dallas Bed Rest Study, which observed that the physical capacity of young men bedridden for three weeks had considerably declined, especially their aerobic capacity. Thirty years later, follow-up on these people actually showed that their aerobic capacity had deteriorated more during those three weeks than after three decades of aging!

BENEFITS OF CARDIAC REHABILITATION FOR PREVENTING POST–HEART ATTACK EVENTS IN CORONARY PATIENTS

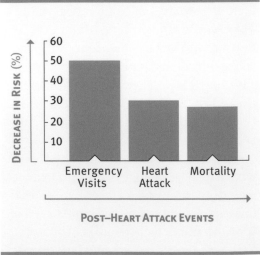

FIGURE 44   Adapted from Nigam and Juneau, 2011.

Example of a Typical Cardiac Rehabilitation and Secondary Prevention Program

Offered by a multidisciplinary team comprising nurses, nutritionists, kinesiologists, and doctors, a cardiac rehabilitation program includes several components. Some programs may also include the services of pharmacists and psychologists.

The first stage involves examining the patient's medical history so as to be able to fully explain to the patient the details of his or her situation: which coronary arteries were affected, which arteries were dilated or bypassed, what kind of stent was used (medicated or not), what the residual function of the heart muscle is (the amount of muscle that remains effective), and the role of each drug prescribed after discharge from the hospital.

Then a treadmill stress test is done to assess exercise capacity, heart rate and blood pressure response, arrhythmias, etc. By means of this test, the "exercise prescription" — the recommended intensity of the activity — is determined.

The kinesiologist uses the results of this stress test to supervise the patient's individualized training.

A nutritionist will do a complete assessment of the individual's dietary habits and propose a Mediterranean diet and practical tools.

Ideally, patients should also follow a stress management program.

A doctor will make any necessary adjustments to the medication to ensure optimal management of risk factors.

A typical cardiac rehabilitation program lasts three months, but obviously patients are advised to continue with these changes for life.

More Intensive Cardiac Rehabilitation

As was mentioned in the preceding chapter, Dr. Dean Ornish's program (www.ornish.com) advocates a similar approach in terms of exercise but instead recommends a vegan diet. Stress management through yoga, meditation, and group sessions is also an essential component of his program. There is no longer any doubt about the results of his approach, which have been published in the best medical journals.

It's now well documented that a physical activity program (cardiac rehabilitation) after a heart attack or operation can not only greatly improve exercise capacity and overall well-being but may also reduce the recurrence of cardiac events (by 25% to 30%), mortality (by 25%), and emergency visits (by 50% in the first year after the attack) (Figure 44). It's therefore strongly recommended to everyone who has had a cardiac event or a cardiac procedure to follow a "cardiac rehabilitation" program. If you have had a heart attack, a cardiac procedure, or heart surgery, ask your doctor about places offering cardiac rehabilitation in your region.

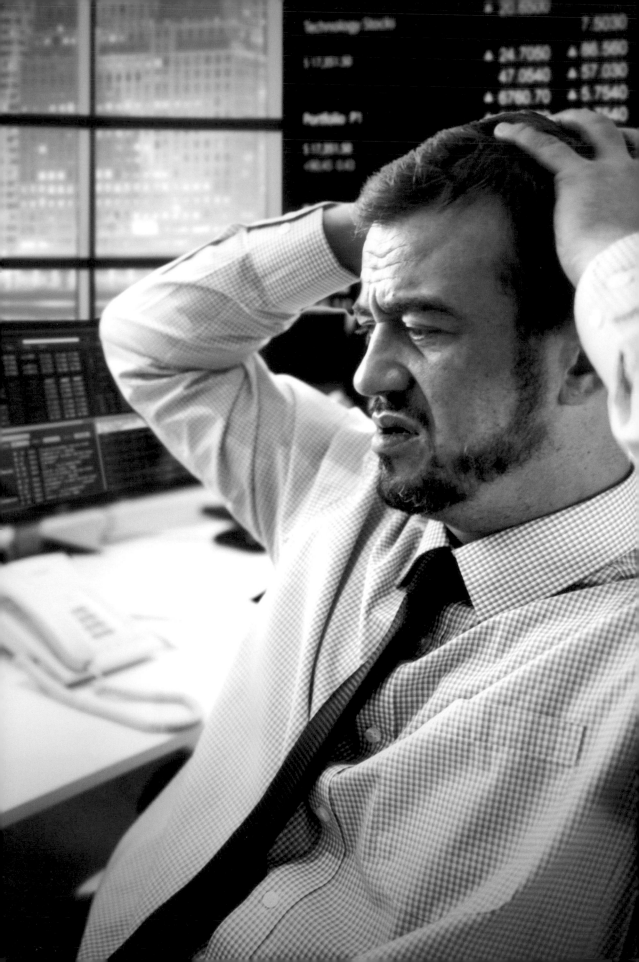

CHAPTER 7

Stress and Heart Disease

In 1942, Dr. Walter B. Cannon, a professor of physiology in the Faculty of Medicine at Harvard University, wrote an article titled "Voodoo Death" that caused a sensation at the time. In great detail, Dr. Cannon described cases of people who died after a severe fright. The stories, originating in various parts of the world, all had certain common traits — the sense or absolute belief that external power wielded by a witch doctor or shaman could cause death and that the victim was powerless to prevent it. Following the publication of Cannon's article, and after many people reported similar experiences, the medical profession figured out what had happened in these cases and managed to explain the mechanisms involved in sudden death during a very stressful event.

A few years later, George L. Engel described eight categories of stressful events capable of causing sudden death:

1. Sudden death of a close person.
2. Very acute grief.
3. Threat of loss of a close person.
4. Anniversary of the death of a close person.
5. Loss of status or self-esteem.
6. Very serious danger or threat.
7. Danger avoided.
8. A happy ending after a tragic event.

For more than 70 years, the connections between the heart and the brain have been thoroughly studied, with over 40,000 articles published on the topic, and the mechanisms involved are now well documented. First, the experience of intense stress has a very significant effect on the autonomic sympathetic nervous system, causing major stimulation of the heart, both directly and by means of hormones, like adrenalin. These changes speed up the heart rate, causing severe

SUDDEN DEATH FOLLOWING JAPAN'S 2011
EARTHQUAKE AND TSUNAMI

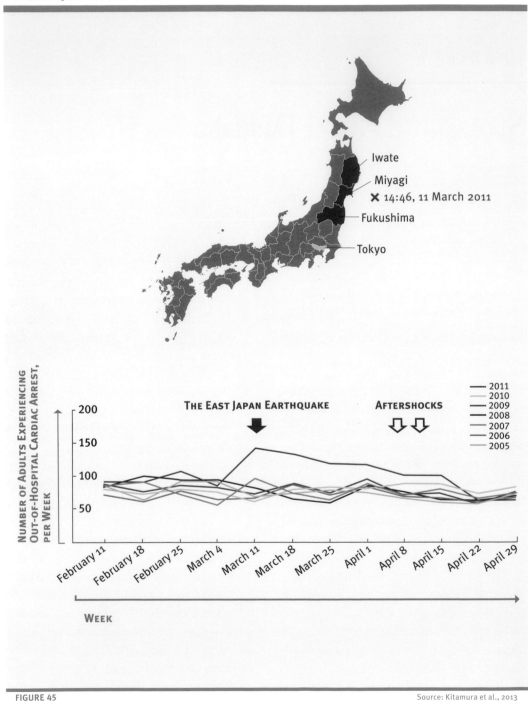

FIGURE 45

Source: Kitamura et al., 2013

arrhythmias or contraction of the coronary arteries. A good example of the negative impact of stress is the considerable increase in sudden death following a tragic event: in the weeks following the earthquake off Sendai and the powerful tsunami that devastated that part of Japan in 2011, the number of people who died suddenly doubled in comparison with preceding years, a trend that continued for three weeks after the initial shock (Figure 45). An increase in sudden death has also been observed after other major earthquakes, showing the extent to which the physiological response to acute stress can have negative repercussions for the heart.

A BROKEN HEART

In the last twenty years, one of the increasingly recognized cardiomyopathies associated with stress is *takotsubo* syndrome, or "broken heart syndrome." First described in 1990 by Japanese cardiologists, this syndrome occurs when someone is exposed to major stress or receives very bad news. This triggers very intense chest pain caused by a heart attack. If the individual survives (which is usually the case), on the patient's arrival at the hospital an acute heart attack will be diagnosed, but without any arterial lesions (no coronary blockages). The name of this syndrome comes from the shape of the left ventricle when it's examined using angiography, since it resembles a *takotsubo*, a trap Japanese fishermen use to catch octopus (Figure 46).

This syndrome is caused by a severe attack in the left ventricle, the part of the heart muscle that pumps arterial blood to the body.

Several triggering factors have been identified over the years, most of them associated with strong negative emotions, like mourning, anger, or fear. Recent results indicate, however, that strong positive emotions (marriage, sports team victory) may also cause this syndrome to occur.

CHRONIC STRESS

Aside from these rather extraordinary examples showing the dramatic effects that the brain and our emotions can have on the heart, thousands of studies have been published on the effect of chronic stress, negative emotions, anxiety, depression, anger, and hostility on the long-term incidence of coronary diseases. In the 1940s and 1950s, the first psychiatrists specializing in "psychosomatic medicine" (usually psychoanalysts) became interested in the psychological characteristics that seemed to be associated with patients suffering from a coronary disease. Later, in the 1960s, two cardiologists, R.H. Rosenman and M. Friedman, described the type A personality, referring to people who are in a rush, impatient, and have difficulty managing their aggressiveness. Having this kind of personality seemed to be related to the development of coronary disease, but this link remains quite controversial today. Research on this subject suggests that it's really two components of the type A personality, anger and hostility, that are major risk factors. A meta-analysis of twenty-five studies has in fact shown that these two emotions are associated with a higher risk for heart attack. They are also related to a higher risk of recurrence, according to nineteen studies done on patients who had already had a cardiac event.

Despite the many observations proving the existence of a link between the brain and cardiovascular disease, this issue remained relatively under the radar until the publication of the INTERHEART Study by Canadian cardiologist Salim Yusuf. Involving nearly twenty-four thousand people in fifty-two different countries, this major study aimed to identify the main heart attack risk factors. Initially, Dr. Yusuf particularly wanted to study classic risk factors, like cholesterol, high blood pressure, abdominal obesity, and

TAKOTSUBO SYNDROME: DYING OF A BROKEN HEART

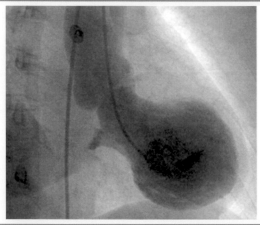 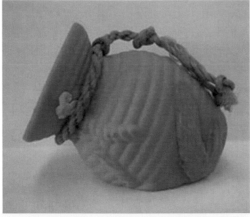

FIGURE 46

Source: Skerrett, 2012

A Case of Heart Attack Caused by Intense Stress (*Takotsubo*)

I myself have had occasion to treat a few cases of *takotsubo* in recent years, and it's always very interesting to realize that acute stress can have such a serious effect on the heart. Recently, I treated a young woman under 30. While she was in a park with her children, she was physically threatened, for no reason at all, by a very aggressive person. Extremely frightened, the young woman fled with her children and, when people offered to help, she collapsed with very intense chest pain. The ambulance brought her immediately to our emergency room, where we diagnosed an acute heart attack in the interior wall of the heart. As in all cases of acute heart attack, the patient was transferred right away to the cardiac catheterization room for an emergency coronary angiography, with the aim of dilating the blocked artery. In this case, there was no blockage and the arteries were in very good shape, with no trace of atherosclerosis. However, when a contrast agent was injected into the left ventricle, the typical vase shape of *takotsubo* syndrome became visible. Luckily, this damage heals well and usually leaves very few after-effects.

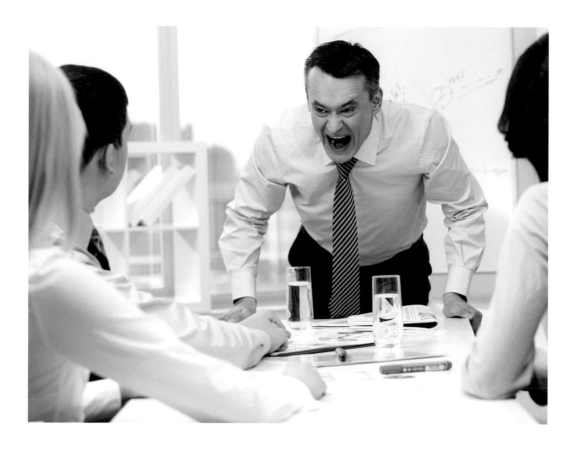

smoking, but, despite his own skepticism, he decided to include in his observations the internal and external stressors perceived by patients. This was a helpful addition, as the study showed that psychosocial stressors are indeed associated with a greater risk of heart attack, and that this effect, although not as significant as that of smoking, is comparable to the effects of hypertension and abdominal obesity. Dr. Yusuf concluded his article by emphasizing that psychosocial factors are much more important than had previously been recognized and that they may contribute to a "substantial" proportion of heart attacks in all societies. Several mechanisms may explain the consequences of stress for the cardiovascular system and, in particular, the coronary arteries: inflammation,

an increase in blood coagulability, and a decrease in fibrinolysis (ability of the blood to dissolve clots), as well as an increase in circulating catecholamines (adrenalin and noradrenalin), which, among other effects, cause the heart to beat faster and increase its contraction strength.

DEPRESSION AND CARDIOVASCULAR DISEASE

As for depression, many studies confirm that a state of depression following a heart attack increases mortality risk in the months after leaving the hospital. A study done at the Montreal Heart Institute by Dr. François Lespérance and his colleagues

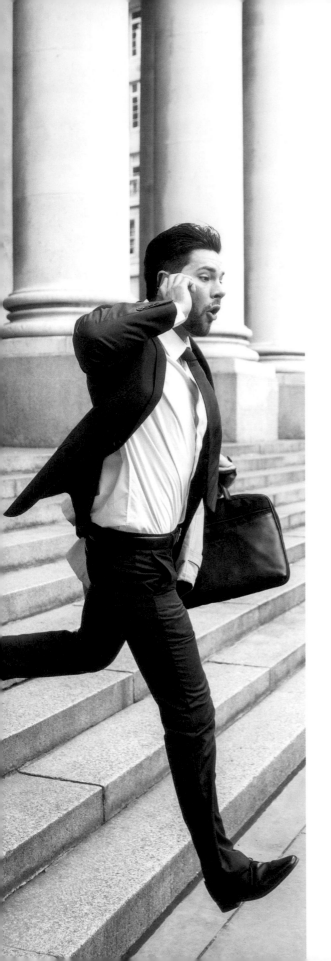

showed that depression arising in patients after being hospitalized for an episode of unstable angina multiplied sixfold the risks of fatal recurrence or heart attack in the year after leaving the hospital.

Although stress and depression are now recognized as major risk factors for cardio-vascular disease, studies on treatments for these conditions using antidepressant or anti-anxiolytic drugs have not produced convincing results. This is a substantial pro-blem, since up to 30% to 40% of patients show depressive symptoms after a heart attack, which can greatly increase the risk of recurrence and premature death if they are not properly treated. A high rate of depression after cardiac surgery has also been noted. At the MHI's EPIC Centre, we have noted for about thirty years that a car-diac rehabilitation program including stress training two or three times a week right at the Centre, in the company of a group of patients in similar circumstances, helps alle-viate depressive feelings and to lower stress considerably after a cardiac event or surgery. When we ask patients what is most impor-tant for them after a heart attack, many of them reply that they would above all like to "lower their stress." Patients also often believe that the stress they are under is the primary cause of their heart condition.

In the early years of my practice, when I asked patients why they kept on smoking, I was surprised to hear "It's all I have left," "It's the only pleasure I have," or "I have a lot of other problems to deal with." It was the same for dietary changes or exercise — "I have other problems to deal with." Answers like this no longer surprise me because I've heard them all so often; they reflect what patients are going through before and after a cardiac event. Behaviours that do not make sense to us (smoking, eating junk food, etc.) are often a source of comfort for people going through difficult situations. Our paternalistic attitude and advice often have no effect on someone with "a lot of other problems to deal with": financial stress, relationship difficulties, loss of self-esteem, concerns about the future, etc. Patients tell us that cigarettes are comforting, alcohol soothes anxiety, junk food helps to make up for all kinds of negative emotions — these are ways they have found to adapt to a difficult situation.

To succeed in effectively preventing recurrence, everything must therefore begin with the brain, because when stress and depressive states are well managed, and priorities have been redefined, patients are prepared to modify their lifestyle habits significantly. Unfortunately, those from socio-economically underprivileged circumstances have problems that medicine alone can do little about; these patients benefit the least from prevention programs, for many economic and social reasons. This situation is well documented in Western countries. Poverty remains the biggest risk factor for premature death.

STRESS MANAGEMENT

How can you change your lifestyle habits when your psychological state is unstable? Based on my experience, the patients with the best outcomes are those who succeed in making quite drastic changes, either by themselves, because the heart attack or cardiac surgery has triggered a reassessment of their personal situation, or with the help of a multidisciplinary team and a stress management program.

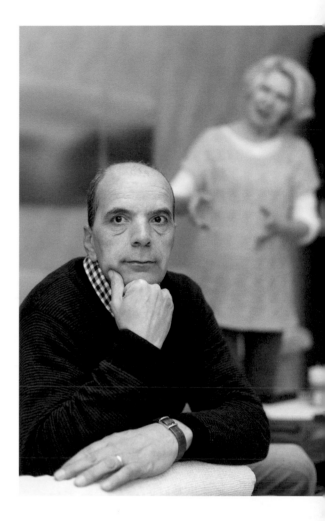

For about ten years, we have been using the approach developed by Jon Kabat-Zinn of the Center for Mindfulness in the Faculty of Medicine at the University of Massachusetts in Boston, an approach called "mindfulness-based stress reduction." This is a fairly intensive approach presented in eight weekly workshops, each 2.5 hours long. This method has proven its value for over 25 years and many scientific articles have demonstrated its effectiveness, not only for reducing stress and improving overall quality of life but also for preventing recurrence after a cardiac event. For

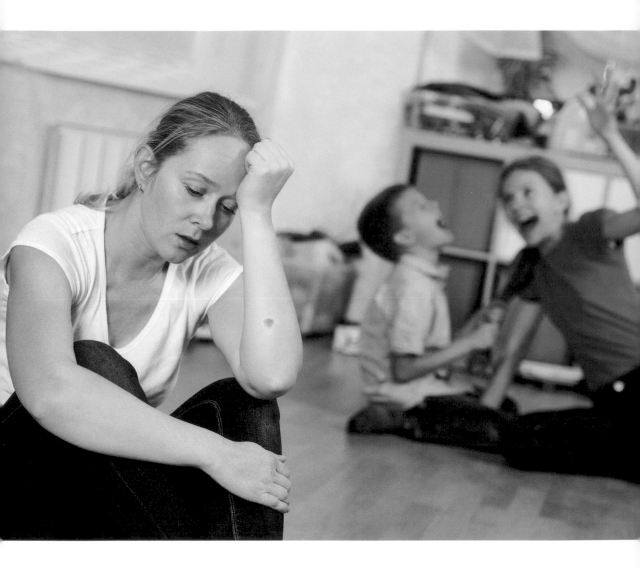

example, a study published in 2012 by R.H. Schneider and his colleagues confirms that practising meditation for twenty minutes twice a day cuts relapses after a cardiac event in half in the five years following. By much better managing their stress, patients more easily adopt all the changes needed to avoid recurrence.

Should this approach also be used in primary prevention, before people become ill? The answer is yes, absolutely. People with many risk factors or who have a mediocre quality of life owing to chronic stress can benefit greatly from the mindfulness-based approach.

What the neurosciences have taught us, and what Rick Hanson describes very well in his book *Hardwiring Happiness* (2013), is that the human brain first went through a "reptilian" stage during evolution, originally reinforcing our reactions to danger to give us a chance at survival. Obviously, the brain evolved and became much more complex with the development of the cerebral

Managing Your Stress — A Few References

At the MHI's EPIC Centre, workshops on stress management through mindfulness are led by Dr. Robert Béliveau and other professionals experienced in this approach. I encourage readers to look into this subject, especially by consulting the following books:

- Jon Kabat-Zinn, *Full Catastrophe Living*
- Rick Hanson, *Hardwiring Happiness*

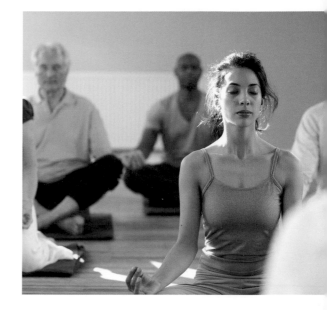

cortex, but traces of our reptilian brain are still there. We therefore have a tendency to view negative events as being three to five times more important than positive ones. For example, Daniel Kahneman, who received the Nobel Prize in Economics in 2002 for his studies on this subject, observed that, given an equal amount of money, a financial loss is much more strongly felt than a gain. In other words, if you lose one thousand dollars on the stock market, the psychological impact will be as powerful as if you had won five thousand dollars. The same holds true for our interpersonal relationships: a negative remark or behaviour directed at us has three to five times more impact than its positive equivalent. This tendency to overemphasize the negative has enabled humans to survive and evolve. For example, worrying and then making sure that there are no snakes hidden in a bush is a situation where the vigilance associated with worry results in avoiding a bite, whereas unconcern in the face of danger can cause death. Our brain is thus programmed to worry. To manage our stress well and improve our quality of life, we have to work actively at "reprogramming" it, so that it gives more weight to the effects of positive experiences than to those of negative ones.

The approach suggested by Jon Kabat-Zinn, Christophe André, and Matthieu Ricard teaches us to take a moment to pause, carefully observe our physical and psychological reactions, and modify our perceptions and behaviours. Contrary to what many people think, meditation is not a relaxation technique, nor a way to hide our problems. Quite the opposite: the goal is to pause briefly, concentrate on the present moment, and observe our thoughts so as to transform the way we think. It's not a means of relaxation, but rather a means of *transformation*.

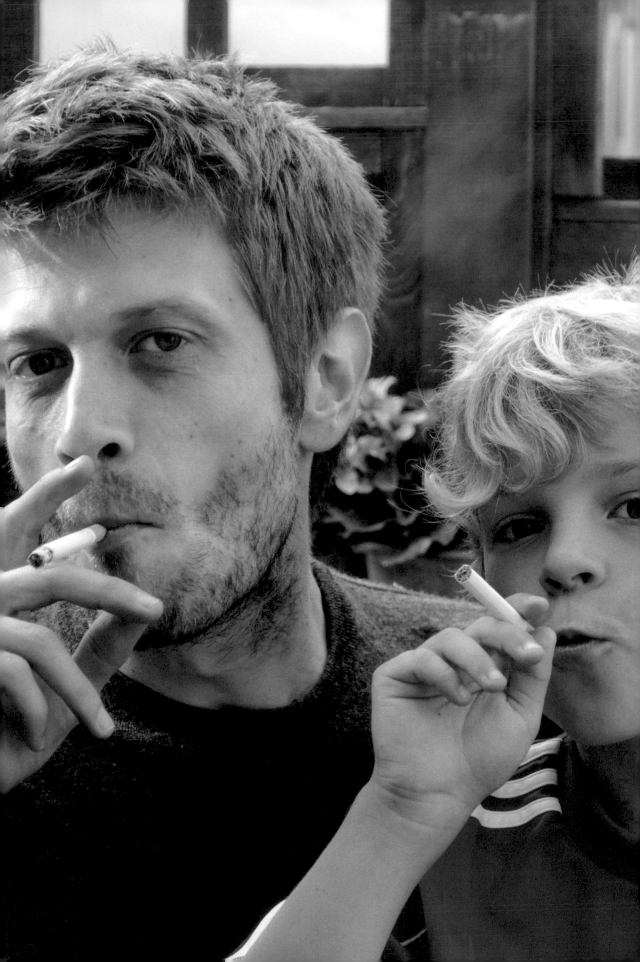

CHAPTER 8

Tobacco and Electronic Cigarettes

According to the latest reports from the World Health Organization and the United States Surgeon General, tobacco use is the biggest cause of "avoidable" mortality in the world. Each year, about six million people die from its effects. Half of regular tobacco consumers will die from their habit; what is less known is that half of these avoidable deaths occur at a relatively young age, between 35 and 69, lowering smokers' life expectancy by 20 to 25 years.

It's believed that in the twentieth century smoking was responsible for no fewer than one hundred million deaths worldwide. If nothing is done to halt its progression, this number will reach one billion in the twenty-first century. In Canada, tobacco causes more than thirty-seven thousand deaths a year, and it's estimated that almost a third of hospital beds are occupied by patients suffering from a tobacco-related illness. These statistics reflect the catastrophic impact of smoking and exposure to second-hand smoke on the entire human body (Figure 47).

TOBACCO AND CARDIOVASCULAR DISEASE

Although we often speak about the major impact of tobacco on the risk of getting lung cancer, remember that cardiovascular disease remains the main cause of death associated with smoking. The risk of having a heart attack increases by 300% in men and 600% in women who smoke twenty cigarettes a day, with the risk being proportional to the number of cigarettes smoked daily. Even those who smoke fewer than five cigarettes a day increase their risk of heart attack. There is therefore no safety threshold where tobacco is concerned.

IMPACT OF TOBACCO AND SECOND-HAND SMOKE ON HEALTH

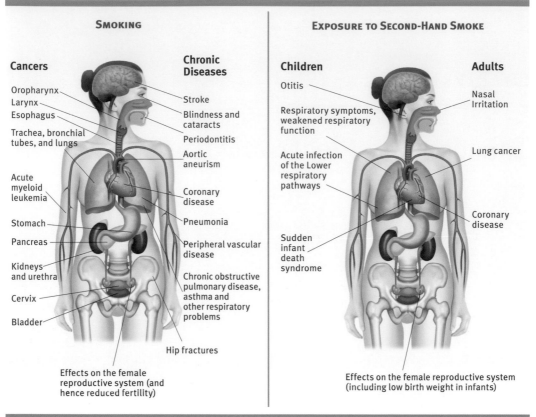

FIGURE 47

Source: Adapted from USDHHS, 2004, 2006

After a coronary artery bypass or a coronary dilation, patients who continue to smoke increase their mortality risk by nearly 70%. Of all the things people can do to improve their cardiovascular health (and their overall health), giving up smoking is beyond any doubt the most important.

SECOND-HAND SMOKE

Unfortunately, even if you do not smoke, regular exposure to secondary smoke (that of smokers) increases your risk of cardiovascular disease (heart attack and stroke) by 20% to 30%. Here too the risk increases with the amount and number of years of exposure. For example, non-smokers married to smokers have a 20% higher risk of having a heart attack and getting lung cancer.

People who live in apartment buildings are also exposed to second-hand smoke from tenants who smoke, since the smoke can penetrate into all the apartments in a building. This is why a number of municipalities in the United States ban smoking in apartment buildings. Smoke-Free Housing Ontario has created a website aiming to promote "smoke-free housing."

TOBACCO CONTROL MEASURES

In 2005, the Quebec government adopted Bill 112, banning smoking in public places. In 2016, Bill 44 came into effect: smoking is now banned on restaurant and bar patios, and in cars when children are present. Ontario banned smoking in all enclosed workplaces and public spaces (including bars and restaurants) in 2006. In every study published on tobacco control measures, it has been noted that in the states or municipalities where regulations and laws like these have been adopted there has been a very significant decline in hospitalizations for tobacco-related diseases. For example, in the city of Kent,

Ohio, the number of admissions for coronary events (heart attack, unstable angina, etc.) dropped by 39% the first year after tobacco control measures were adopted and by 47% after three years. In Olmstead county, Minnesota, the incidence of sudden death decreased by 17% in the eighteen months following the implementation of laws banning smoking in restaurants and workplaces.

QUITTING SMOKING HAS ALMOST IMMEDIATE BENEFITS

The reduction in mortality observed very soon after a simple ban on smoking in public places shows how quickly a decrease in smoking leads to improvement in health. It's never too late to stop smoking, since doing so at any age substantially reduces disease risk, especially for cardiovascular disease:

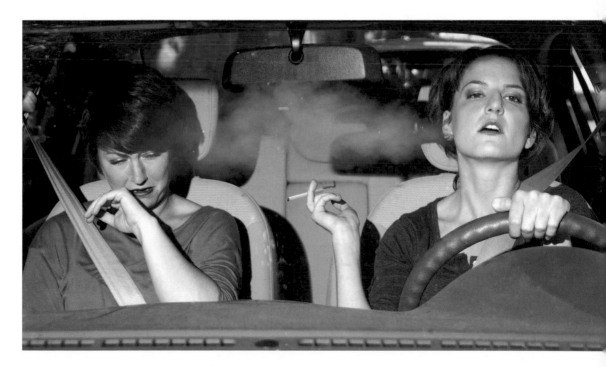

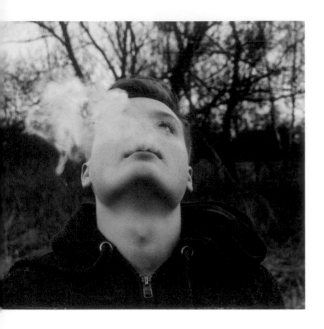

- Twenty minutes after the last cigarette, blood pressure and heart rate return to normal.
- Eight hours later, the risk of coronary artery spasm is almost eliminated.
- Twenty-four hours later, the levels of carbon monoxide and circulating catecholamines (which stimulate the heart) return to normal.
- In the first year, patients who stop smoking after a heart attack reduce their risk of recurrence by 50%, and their risk of stroke is similar to someone who has never smoked.
- After five years, the risk of a coronary event (heart attack, sudden death) is similar to that of a non-smoker.

No other medical or surgical intervention is as effective for cardiovascular health as quitting smoking. Furthermore, it's the least expensive. It's therefore surprising that more hospitals do not offer a smoking treatment program for hospitalized patients. At the Montreal Heart Institute, this kind of program is offered to all patients, funded by our foundation. Similar programs are offered at the University of Ottawa Heart Institute, and through the Nicotine Dependence Clinic at the Centre for Addiction and Mental Health (CAMH) in Toronto.

In general, regardless of the disease (cancer, respiratory illness, or cardiovascular disease), experts agree that quitting smoking increases life expectancy by ten years. Obviously, the sooner you quit, the greater the benefits.

In addition to adding years, quality of life is definitely improved by quitting smoking. The coughing, breathlessness, recurring respiratory infections, and loss of taste that result from smoking are harmful symptoms that quickly disappear when you stop.

HOW TO QUIT SMOKING SUCCESSFULLY

Studies show that it's very hard to stop smoking without help: barely 5% of those who try manage to still be non-smokers after one year. However, this success rate can easily be increased by 20% or 25% by means of an assistance program combined with pharmacological treatments (Figure 48).

Smoking cessation support programs are usually run by a nurse, who can advise the smoker, prescribe medication under a doctor's supervision, check tolerance to medications and their side effects, and offer psychological support in person and by means of regular telephone follow-up.

ELECTRONIC CIGARETTES: A SOLUTION OR A NEW PROBLEM?

First, we should note that it's the hundreds of combustion products in tobacco cigarettes that cause health problems, not the nicotine. The latter is a drug that rapidly creates a dependency that makes you smoke, but it is not responsible for cardiovascular diseases, nor for lung cancer: "You smoke for the nicotine, but you die from tobacco." Nicotine replacement products, like gums and nicotine patches, have been used for more than 20 years and studies show they are very safe. There are also nicotine inhalers and vaporizers that have been proven harmless.

Electronic cigarettes (e-cigarettes: see Figure 49) contain water, plant glycerin, propylene glycol, flavouring, and nicotine in varying concentrations. Invented by a Chinese pharmacist in 2003, they appeared in Europe in 2007. The British and French thus have more than nine years of experience with this technological innovation. The first generations of e-cigarettes were of poor quality, but, as with all technology, the new disposable or refillable models are much more effective: better batteries, more reliable atomizers, etc. Despite this progress, e-cigarettes are nowhere near as effective as tobacco cigarettes for delivering nicotine to the brain. This is why heavy smokers (those who smoke more than a pack a day) are seldom satisfied by the nicotine dose delivered in every inhalation.

First, there is a big difference in heat between the two products: the combustion temperature at the tip of a tobacco cigarette is almost 900°C, as opposed to about 80°C for an e-cigarette, which does not produce combustion (nothing burns), but rather a vapour that is actually a spray of fine droplets in suspension. E-cigarettes do not release carbon monoxide, nor fine particles, nor obviously the 4,000 combustion products found in tobacco cigarette smoke. Analyses of various kinds of e-cigarettes show they contain in general from ten to four hundred times fewer harmful products than tobacco cigarettes. While e-cigarettes are certainly not ideal, nor without risk, most experts agree they are much less harmful than tobacco.

In 2007, England's Royal College of Physicians had already expressed this opinion, and in April 2016, it published a very thorough update with more than 600 scientific references. In this recent report, the College reaffirmed: "Although it is not possible to quantify the long-term health risks associated with e-cigarettes precisely, the available data suggest that they are unlikely to exceed 5% of those associated with smoked tobacco products, and may well be substantially lower than this figure."

As for the effectiveness of e-cigarettes in helping people to stop smoking, the various findings published to date indicate that the figures vary from 50% to 70%. Dr. Gaston Ostiguy, a pulmonologist at the McGill University Health Centre (MUHC) and a pioneer in the fight against smoking in Quebec, reports a success level of 50% in especially hard-to-treat patients. Some of his patients with chronic pulmonary diseases are extremely dependent on tobacco and continue to smoke despite many severe symptoms (persistent coughing, frequent respiratory infections, noticeable shortness of breath after minimal effort, etc.). This is a long way from the occasional social smoker! These patients have "tried everything,"

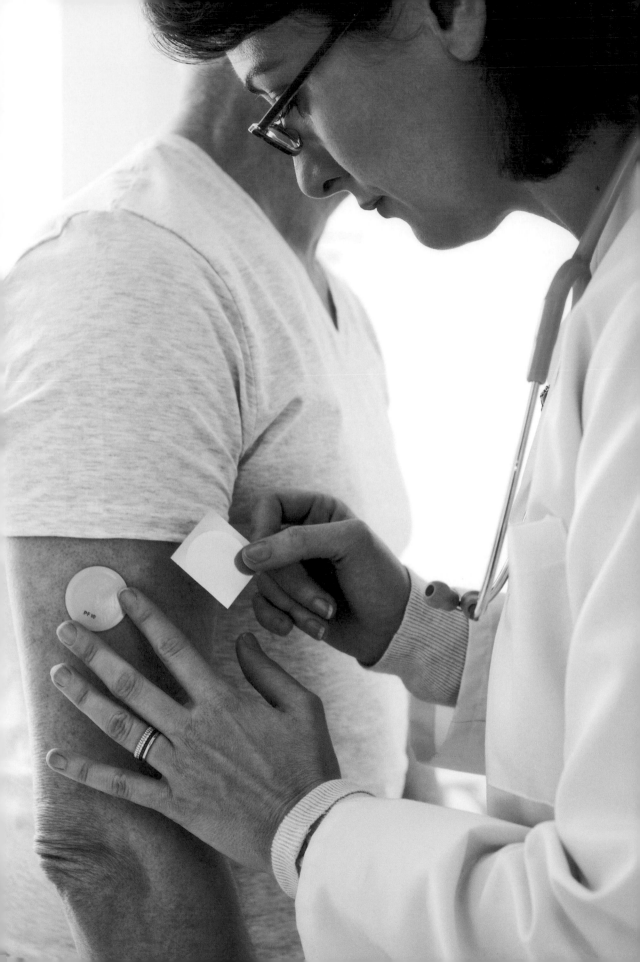

without success, and a success level of 50% maintained for a year is more than twice that of conventional pharmaceutical methods.

At the EPIC Centre's smoking treatment clinic at the MHI, we suggest e-cigarettes to smokers who have experienced nothing but failure using recognized pharmacological methods. With these patients, our success rate is about 70%. It must be emphasized that most of our heart patients appear to be less "hooked" on cigarettes than do those with pulmonary diseases. Since 2013, having learned from my European cardiologist and tobacco addiction specialist colleagues how effective this method has been, I have been suggesting e-cigarettes to my heart patients who smoke to help them quit.

Several official bodies in Canada and the United States are still fiercely opposed to e-cigarettes because they fear that it "renormalizes" the act of smoking and, especially, that it encourages teenagers. I fully understand their concerns, but I do not share them, as this is not at all what the British and French data show. In both countries, tobacco cigarette use has continued to decrease among young people since the advent of e-cigarettes. For French teenagers, tobacco cigarettes have become "old-fashioned." Little by little, British and French specialists have understood that this is a technological innovation with the potential to reduce smoking among young people and not the opposite. Public Health England repeated this position statement in a report, *E-cigarettes, an evidence update*, published in August 2015. The Office français de prévention du tabagisme (OFT, the French smoking prevention agency) also produced an extensive report, *La cigarette électronique et les jeunes*, in the same vein in 2014. The first paragraph of the document affirms that the electronic cigarette increasingly appears to act as a *smoking cessation product on both an individual and a collective level* as shown by French and English data, from the two countries where e-cigarettes are readily available (while in Belgium, for example, where the sale of e-liquid is forbidden, smoking rates and cigarette sales have increased).

On our side of the Atlantic, public health specialists overall remain very opposed to e-cigarettes and refuse to believe they have benefits. I understand that when you have fought for 50 years

SMOKING CESSATION RATES COMPARED AFTER ONE YEAR

Long-term smoking cessation rates are higher when both drug therapy and behavioural support are offered.	No Therapy	Counselling	Behavioural Therapy
No Medication or Placebo	5%	10%	15%
Medication	10%	20%	30%

FIGURE 48

against tobacco cigarettes, it's difficult to accept anything that seems to resemble them. I am convinced that there is also among Americans and Canadians a slightly puritanical and moralizing side that is less common in Europe. We have difficulty, for example, replacing "one dependency for another," whereas, in practice, nicotine dependency is quite harmless, without the damage associated with tobacco combustion. Many ex-smokers consume nicotine gum for years without noticing any negative effect on their health.

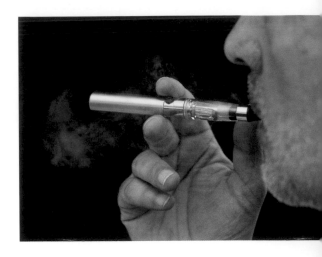

My patients who have stopped smoking thanks to e-cigarettes have usually quit using them after a year, without going back to tobacco. Often, those who like the "act" of smoking keep on with the e-cigarette, but without nicotine. In addition, nicotine without tobacco seems to cause less dependency, since most users reduce their nicotine concentration over time, instead of increasing it. These data are well documented. Dr. Karl Olov Fagerström, one of the best-known nicotine dependency experts in the world, who invented the well-known questionnaire named after him, also affirms that data gathered to date show that nicotine alone creates less dependency than when it's combined with tobacco. Among the 4,000 combustion products in tobacco cigarettes, there are undoubtedly some that increase nicotine dependency. We know that cigarette manufacturers add many chemical products to tobacco with the aim of making the smoke "milder" and increasing dependency. Adding sugars,

ELECTRONIC CIGARETTES

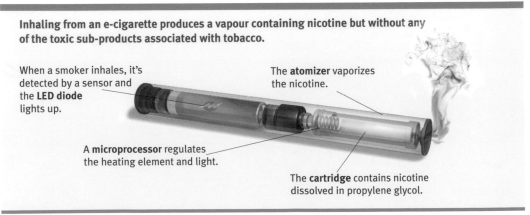

Inhaling from an e-cigarette produces a vapour containing nicotine but without any of the toxic sub-products associated with tobacco.

When a smoker inhales, it's detected by a sensor and the **LED diode** lights up.

The **atomizer** vaporizes the nicotine.

A **microprocessor** regulates the heating element and light.

The **cartridge** contains nicotine dissolved in propylene glycol.

FIGURE 49

for example, gives a milder taste and produces, during combustion, monoamine oxidase inhibitors, which increase dopamine levels and, as a result, tobacco dependency.

In conclusion, if you smoke, your priority, in terms of prevention, is to quit. If you are heavily dependent on cigarettes, you will greatly increase your chances of success by consulting a smoking cessation centre or a specialized clinic. If you have tried all the medications available on the market without success, e-cigarettes may prove to be an effective solution.

A Book on E-Cigarettes

For further information, I recommend *Electronic Cigarettes: A Briefing for Stop Smoking Services*, by A. McEwen and H. McRobbie, produced in 2016 by the National Centre for Smoking Cessation and Training (NCSCT), in partnership with Public Health England.

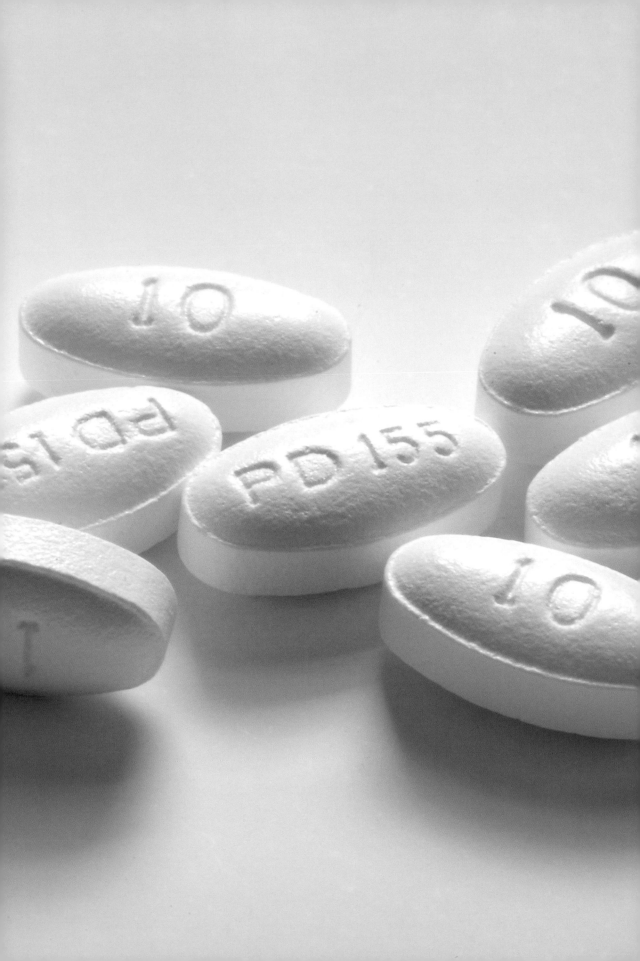

CHAPTER 9

Statins in Primary and Secondary Prevention

Blaming cholesterol for the development of atheromatous plaques led to a veritable race against the clock to discover drugs that would lower LDL cholesterol levels and, in doing so, reduce the risk of cardiovascular disease. The discovery of a new class of drugs able to block cholesterol production by the liver completely changed the medical approach to cardiovascular disease prevention. These drugs are called statins.

FROM MOULD TO MEDICINE

Statins would likely never have seen the light of day without the persistence of Japanese biochemist Akira Endo. A great admirer of Alexander Fleming, who had shown that certain kinds of mould produced antibiotic substances like penicillin to protect themselves from bacteria in their environment, Dr. Endo put forward the hypothesis that micro-organisms could also defend themselves by secreting substances able to hinder the formation of cholesterol and its derivatives, which are absolutely essential for the survival of many microbes. To identify these molecules, his team cultivated nearly six thousand strains of various micro-organisms. The anti-cholesterol potential of each one was examined by measuring its ability to block the activity of *HMG-CoA reductase*, the most important of the thirty or so enzymes that work together to change acetate into cholesterol.

It was a lengthy task, but they were eventually able to show that the mould *Penicillium citrinum* did indeed produce a substance that inhibited the activity of *HMG-CoA reductase*, a molecule they called "mevastatin" to emphasize its ability to block ("stat," derived from "static") the synthesis of mevalonate. A few years later, a very similar molecule, lovastatin, found naturally in some mushrooms (oyster mushrooms) and yeasts (red rice yeast) was produced on a large scale by the Merck company and put on the market in 1987 under the name Mevacor to treat hypercholesterolemia. Thus was born the "great family of statins" and, with the arrival on the market of many derivatives (simvastatin, atorvastatin, etc.), it has become one of the most widely sold drug classes in the world. After having played an exceptionally important role in treatments for infectious diseases by means of penicillin, *Penicillium* have, 50 years later, revolutionized cardiology through statins, making these moulds the most profitable micro-organisms in the history of the pharmaceutical industry!

PREVENTING RECURRENCE

The clinical importance of statins is well illustrated in studies on *secondary* prevention, when the drug is given to patients with coronary disease, including those who have already had a heart attack or who have been hospitalized for unstable angina, as well as those who have undergone angioplasty or coronary aortic bypasses. People with stable angina or those who have received a diagnosis of coronary disease following an examination, like a stress test using nuclear medicine or a stress ultrasound, also benefit from this treatment. All patients who have a coronary disease run the risk of seeing their disease progress and having a recurrence or a worsening of their angina symptoms. Many studies indicate that statins reduce significantly the likelihood of experiencing another cardiac event (Figure 50).

The publication of the famous 4S Study of 4,444 Scandinavian patients at the beginning of the 1990s showed the effectiveness of one statin, simvastatin, in coronary patients. This study showed that 11.5% of untreated patients (the placebo group) died after a little more than five years, compared with 8.2% of those treated with the statin. There was therefore a 4% reduction in absolute risk of mortality, equal to a relative risk reduction of 28.6% (3.3% divided by 11.5% = 0.29). As for the incidence of heart attacks, there were 502 in the placebo group (22.6%) and 353 15.6%) in the group treated with the statin, for an absolute reduction of 6.7%, which gives a relative reduction of 29.6% (6.7% divided by 22.6% = 29.6%). As Figure 50 shows, similar results have also been obtained in other studies on *secondary* prevention, and it has now been clearly established that treating patients who have had a cardiac event helps prevent recurrence and even death. As a result, these medications are now part of the standard therapeutic arsenal for treating anyone who has survived a cardiac event or has a stable coronary disease.

It's important, however, to realize that statins' protective effect, even though well proven, is not a panacea, since the absolute risk reduction is modest (Figure 50) and patients remain at high risk.

Risk that remains high in spite of treatment is called "residual risk" by cardiology researchers. It is also observed when higher doses of a more powerful statin are administered and the LDL cholesterol level is clearly lowered, to about 1.6 mmol/L. In my view, one of the best illustrations of this is the PROVE IT Study, published in the *New England Journal of Medicine* in 2004. This study examined the effectiveness of

IMPACT OF STATINS ON THE PREVENTION OF MORTALITY AND CORONARY EVENTS IN PATIENTS ALREADY AFFECTED BY HEART DISEASE (SECONDARY PREVENTION)

For comparison purposes, the impact of diet (Lyon Study) is indicated

Study	Parameters Measured	Placebo Group	Statin Group	Relative Risk Reduction	Absolute Risk Reduction
4S	Total Mortality	11.5%	8.2%	28.6%	4%
	Major Cardiovascular Events	22.6%	15.6%	29.6%	6.7%
CARE	Mortality from Cardiovascular Disease	5.7%	4.6%	19%	1.1%
	Fatal and Non-Fatal Heart Attacks	13.2%	10.2%	23%	3.0%
LIPID	Total Mortality	14.1%	11%	22%	3.1%
	Heart Attack	10.3%	7.4%	28%	2.9%
HPS	Total Mortality	14.7%	12.9%	12%	1.8%
	Mortality from Coronary Disease	6.9%	5.7%	19%	1.3%
		AHA Diet (Low-Fat)	Mediterranean Diet		
Lyon Study (Mediterranean Diet)	Total Mortality	11.7%	6.4%	45%	5.3%
	Mortality from Coronary Disease	9.3%	2.7%	71%	6.6%
	Fatal and Non-Fatal Heart Attacks	12.2%	3.6%	70%	8.6%

FIGURE 50

two statins in preventing recurrence and mortality after a cardiac event — atorvastatin, in a dose of 80 milligrams per day, and pravastatin, in a dose of 40 milligrams per day. After 30 months, the researchers reported a much greater decrease in LDL cholesterol with atorvastatin, as one might have expected, given the drug's powerful hypocholesterolemic effect (Figure 51A). The more significant drop in LDL cholesterol in the group treated with atorvastatin was accompanied by a reduction in recurrence of cardiac events of 3.9% (26.3% compared with 22.4%), compared with the pravastatin group, whose LDL cholesterol decreased less. What is important to note is that the incidence of mortality and major cardiovascular events after thirty months of treatment remained very high, *at* 22.4%, even in the group whose LDL cholesterol decreased to 1.6 mmol/L (Figure 51B). In other words, even when treatment with a maximum dose of statin results in a marked reduction in blood LDL cholesterol, there is still a significant percentage of patients (almost a quarter in this case) who remain at very high risk of recurrence in the three years following the beginning of treatment.

Can this residual risk be lowered and the survival chances of coronary patients be increased? As is often the case, efforts in this direction are mainly devoted to the discovery of medications able to lower LDL cholesterol levels even further. However, results to date are not very conclusive. For example, combining a statin with a molecule that reduces cholesterol absorption in the intestine (ezetimibe) leads to an additional decrease in LDL cholesterol (to 1.4 mmol/L on average, or well below levels considered

desirable). In the IMPROVE-IT study, the decrease in serious events is only 2% (34.7% compared with 32.7%), a rather weak effect, even though it is statistically significant. Furthermore, there is no difference at all in the total mortality rate between the two groups (15.3% compared to 15.4%) and the mortality rate due to cardiovascular disease (6.8% compared with 6.9%). These results have been judged insufficiently convincing by the consultative committee of the American Food and Drug Administration (FDA), which therefore does not advise the use of this medication in combination with a statin in coronary patients.

Is there a combination of medications that will one day make it possible to lower LDL cholesterol levels more dramatically and markedly reduce rates of mortality caused by cardiovascular disease? We will have to wait for the results of ongoing clinical studies on PCSK9 inhibitors, a new class of drugs that reduce cholesterol significantly, to be able to answer that question. When they are taken with statins, these inhibitors do indeed spectacularly lower LDL cholesterol (from 50% to 70%) and should therefore, in theory, considerably improve the survival of patients at high risk of mortality from cardiovascular disease. However, if these medications do prove effective, we should expect their use to be strictly controlled in order to limit costs to the healthcare system, since they are extremely expensive (about $7,000 per person per year in Canada but $14,000 in the United States).

The search for new drugs able to improve the survival chances of patients with cardiovascular disease must not, however, make us forget that diet, physical activity, and stress management are

THE PROVE-IT STUDY: COMPARISON OF THE EFFECTIVENESS OF TWO STATINS IN PREVENTING RECURRENCE AND MORTALITY AFTER A CORONARY EVENT

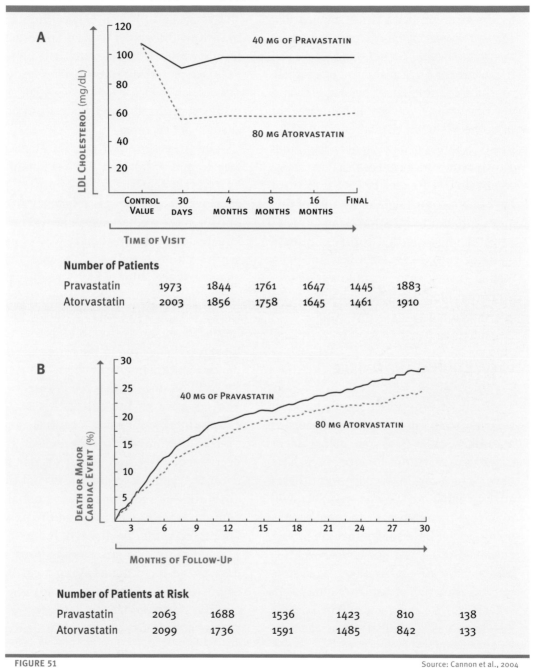

Number of Patients

Pravastatin	1973	1844	1761	1647	1445	1883
Atorvastatin	2003	1856	1758	1645	1461	1910

Number of Patients at Risk

Pravastatin	2063	1688	1536	1423	810	138
Atorvastatin	2099	1736	1591	1485	842	133

FIGURE 51

Source: Cannon et al., 2004

effective and inexpensive ways of greatly decreasing the risk of recurrence. Results of the Lyon Heart Study, in which subjects were prescribed a Mediterranean diet, showed *a reduction in recurrence risk twice that of statins* (see Chapter 5 and Figure 50). If you have had a cardiac event or a cardiac procedure (angioplasty, bypass, etc.) and you take statins, you should be aware that it has been shown that adopting healthy lifestyle habits *in addition to taking statins* greatly reduces recurrence risk. Two major recent studies directed by Dr. Salim Yusuf have again confirmed the validity of this approach, not to mention Dean Ornish's research showing that coronary disease could be completely stabilized and even made to *regress* through an intensive program that modifies lifestyle habits, as we saw in Chapter 5.

PREVENTION AT THE SOURCE

The limits of an approach strictly based on the use of statins to reduce mortality related to cardiovascular disease are more evident in *primary* prevention, for people who have never had a cardiovascular event (heart attack, angina, etc.) or who are not known to have coronary disease. In these people, many studies have shown that the impact of these drugs on serious cardiac events is quite small, and most have observed an absolute risk reduction of just 1% (Figure 52). In other words, for every one hundred people who take the drug daily for years, *only one* will be saved from having a coronary event.

How is it then that statins have acquired the reputation of being indispensable for the primary prevention of cardiovascular disease and rank among the most

commonly prescribed drugs? There are several reasons for this, the main one being of course that our Western medical culture always favours a pharmacological approach in treating diseases. If the LDL cholesterol level is even slightly elevated, the preference is to prescribe a statin as a precaution, rather than to tackle the causes, such as a mediocre-quality diet and a lack of physical exercise, for example.

The great popularity of statins in *primary* prevention can also be explained by the fact that their weak impact on cardiovascular events is relatively little known in the medical community. This is largely due to the customary way of presenting clinical studies by showing only *relative* risk reduction, which amplifies the perception of statins' protective effect. A good example is the ASCOT Study, which helped make atorvastatin (Lipitor) the most profitable drug in the history of the pharmaceutical industry, with revenues of $140 billion since it appeared in 1996.

As Figure 52 indicates, this statin causes the risk of having a cardiac event to decline from 3% to 1.9%, which is a decrease of only 1.1% in *absolute* risk for coronary events. Except that it is not this absolute risk reduction that is usually communicated to doctors and the population, but rather *relative* risk reduction, a much more dramatic way to present data. Since the risk of having a cardiac event when not taking any drugs is 3% and the statin reduces this risk to 1.9%, the authors of the study conclude, correctly, that the statin reduces the risk of heart attack by 36%. The calculation is as follows: 1.1%, representing the reduction in risk (the difference between the percentages in the two groups), is divided by 3%,

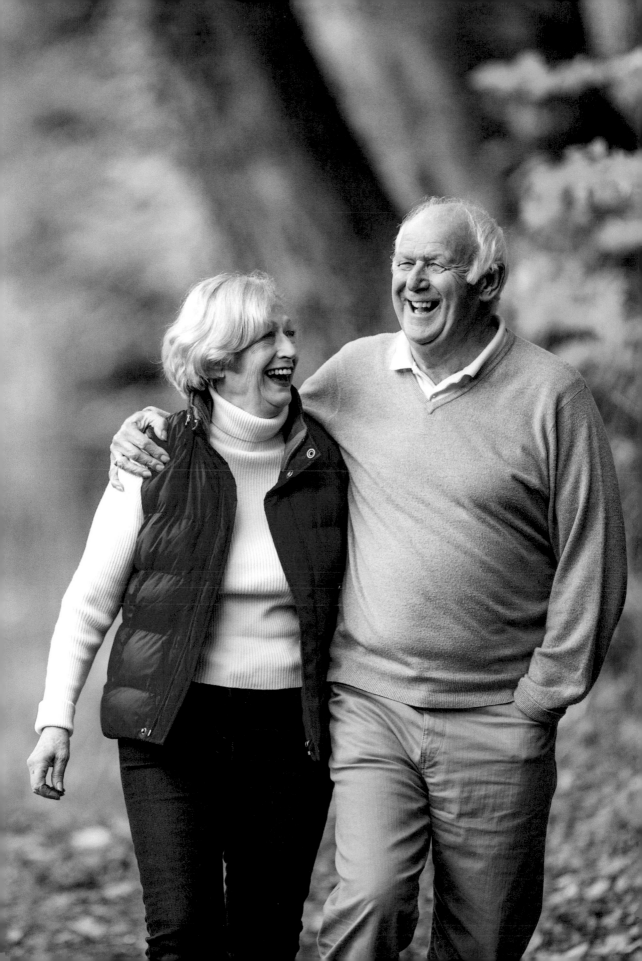

IMPACT OF STATINS ON THE PREVENTION OF MORTALITY AND CORONARY EVENTS IN THE POPULATION (PRIMARY PREVENTION)

Study	Parameters Measured	Placebo Group	Statin Group	Relative Risk Reduction	Absolute Risk Reduction
WOSCOPS	Total Mortality	4.1 %	3.2 %	22 %	0.9 %
	Mortality from Coronary Disease	1.7 %	1.2 %	29 %	0.5 %
	Non-Fatal Heart Attacks	6.5 %	4.6 %	29 %	1.9 %
ASCOT	Total Mortality	4.1 %	3.6 %	12 %	0.5 %
	Fatal and Non-Fatal Heart Attacks	3.0 %	1.9 %	36 %	1.1 %
AFCAPS	Mortality from Cardiovascular Disease	0.7 %	0.5 %	28 %	0.2 %
	Major Strokes	5.5 %	3.5 %	36 %	2 %
ALLHAT	Total Mortality	15.3 %	14.9 %	2.6 %	0.4 %
	Fatal and Non-Fatal Heart Attacks	10.4 %	9.3 %	10 %	1.1 %
HOPE-3	Mortality from Cardiovascular Disease	2.7 %	2.4 %	11 %	0.3 %
	Severe Strokes	4.8 %	3.7 %	23 %	1.1 %
		Standard Low-Fat Diet	Mediterranean Diet High in Extra-Virgin Olive Oil		
PREDIMED (Mediterranean Diet)	Heart Attack, Stroke, and Mortality from Cardiovascular Disease	4.4 %	3.7 %	16 %	0.7 %

FIGURE 52

the risk of cardiac events in the placebo group, which gives 36% (1.1 divided by 3 = 0.36, or 36%). All the publicity concerning Lipitor (Figure 53) in medical journals is based on the promise that the statin can decrease by more than a third the risk of heart attack.

However, when it's explained to doctors and patients that the absolute risk is really only reduced by 1.1%, they are less enthusiastic.

More recently, in April 2016, the HOPE-3 Study again showed a 1% decrease in cardiac events (4.8% compared with 3.7%) with a statin, rosuvastatin, but the headlines once again highlighted the 23% decrease in relative risk (4.8 – 3.7 = 1.1 and 1.1 divided by 4.8 = 23%). In addition, the table of results shows that mortality is no lower in the group treated with this drug. In reference to this study, cardiologist John Mandrola wrote in his blog on the Internet medical site Medscape that his biggest concern was that doctors might be making the mistake of prescribing a drug when walking and eating well would be more effective.

In June 2016, a study published in a British medical journal showed that many people had stopped taking statins for primary prevention following the publication of newspaper articles criticizing these drugs. For many cardiologists, me included, this is not a catastrophe, since their effectiveness is not very significant in primary prevention. Dr. Eric Topol, one of the most influential cardiologists on the planet, commented on this study in a popular magazine in the United States: "For primary prevention, we have too many people taking statins unnecessarily — they have a small benefit of about two per one hundred people."

WHAT SHOULD YOU DO IF YOUR DOCTOR RECOMMENDS A STATIN?

In some cases, there is no doubt that taking a statin may be a good choice in *primary* prevention, for example if you have a genetic disease called familial hypercholesterolemia or you have several risk factors (hereditary early coronary disease, high blood pressure, diabetes, abdominal obesity, elevated cholesterol). This makes you very likely to experience a cardiovascular event and your doctor will insist on prescribing a statin. The more risk factors you accumulate, the more useful the statin will be. Remember, however, that if you do not change your lifestyle, the statin will have only a very limited effect, an absolute risk reduction of about 1%, as mentioned earlier. You will thus not really be protected from a cardiovascular event, and I would therefore strongly advise you to adopt a very different lifestyle. If you decide to do so, you will be much better protected than if you just take a drug.

Some doctors recommend statins to healthy people if their LDL cholesterol is

LIPITOR

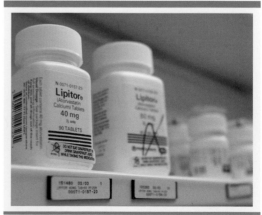

FIGURE 53

above the values deemed normal. As we saw in Chapter 3, the risk of cardiovascular disease is determined largely based on age and laboratory values, whereas body weight, waist circumference, dietary habits, and frequency of physical activity are simply not taken into account, which is absurd. If you have no other cardiovascular disease risk factors, there is no history of cardiovascular disease in your immediate family (father, mother, siblings), you do not smoke, you do not have high blood pressure or diabetes, and only your LDL cholesterol level is elevated, it's completely reasonable not to take statins if you modify your diet and get enough exercise. As with all important health issues, the pros and cons of a new drug prescription or any medical intervention must be discussed with your doctor. It's a question of making a well-informed decision for you, based on available scientific data and your own values. Consider your long-term risk and ask yourself if you want to take a medication for the rest of your life to reduce the risk of cardiovascular disease by about 1%. If the answer is no, do you believe yourself capable of profoundly changing your lifestyle habits and are you motivated to do so? As we have seen in the previous chapters, changing habits is much more effective, and at the same time you will improve your quality of life.

SIDE EFFECTS OF STATINS

For people at low risk of having a coronary event, a "moderate" approach in terms of statins is especially advisable since these drugs can have side effects that cause muscular problems. For a long time, the extent of these undesirable effects was downplayed, on the pretext that they were very uncommon in clinical studies, but today we know that their incidence is much higher in the general population. This is explained by the fact that large-scale clinical studies are financed by the pharmaceutical industry. Participants are rigorously selected so as to eliminate, before the trials even begin, those who do not tolerate the drug.

The most common side effects are generally experienced in the leg muscles, as pain and weakness, but may also affect the arm muscles in people who do physical labour or play sports using their arms. Some people tolerate this discomfort quite well, but about 10% to 15% of patients find it really hard to put up with, which often results in their abandoning the treatment outright. In addition, half of patients stop their statin treatment by themselves during the first year.

Studies have also shown that statins cause exercise intolerance, meaning that people who take these drugs find exercise more difficult. Several studies have shown that statins had a significant effect on the muscles and could even reduce the benefits of fitness training. For example, Catherine Mikus and her team published a study on this subject in the *Journal of the American College of Cardiology* in 2013. Thirty-seven participants were divided randomly into two groups. All the participants had to exercise while taking either a statin (first group) or a placebo (second group). After 12 weeks of supervised training, researchers noted that the maximum aerobic capacity (maximal oxygen consumption) of patients in the first group had not increased. On the other hand, in the group that took the

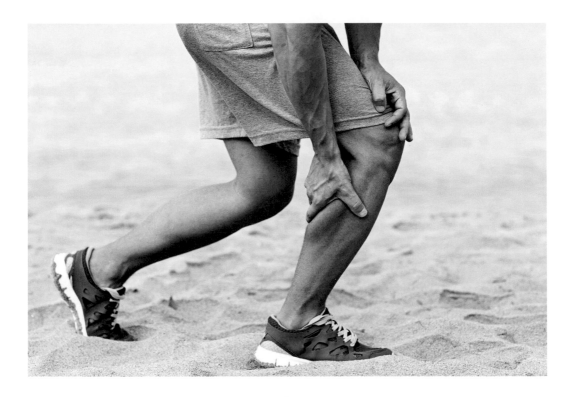

placebo, there was a completely normal increase in maximal oxygen consumption, as is always observed after this kind of program. In other words, the statin had the effect of blocking the beneficial effect of training on exercise capacity.

To shed light on why this happened, researchers did muscle biopsies in both groups and could see that levels of an important muscle enzyme, *citrate synthase*, were much lower in people taking the statin. This enzyme plays an important role in the functioning of mitochondria, the cells' "power plant," suggesting that statins partially prevent the muscle from generating the energy needed for exertion. Similar results have been reported by several authors, clearly showing that when someone complains of exercise intolerance, this is not a purely subjective

impression; there is a physiological reason for it. These side effects, like muscle aches, disappear completely when the medication is stopped.

When this situation occurs in one of my patients, I first check to see whether stopping the statin for two or three weeks eliminates the symptoms. If so, another statin can be tried in the hope it will be better tolerated. Unfortunately, the symptoms usually come back and stopping the treatment permanently must be considered if the discomfort is intolerable. In these very specific cases, I advise patients to stop the drug, but I explain that they absolutely have to change their lifestyle habits, since they will no longer benefit from statin protection, weak though it is.

Many patients are very concerned when they stop taking their statin because

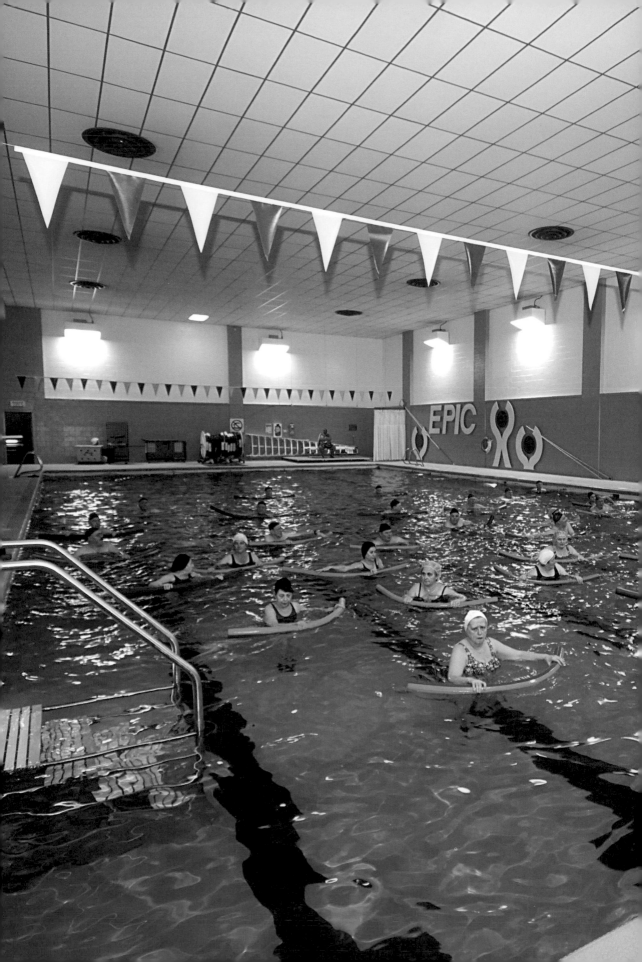

of intolerable side effects. It's nonetheless important to remember that by profoundly changing your lifestyle, you can more than make up for the statin's beneficial effect.

A HOLISTIC APPROACH

As we saw in chapters 2 and 3, the formation of atheromatous plaques is an extremely complex process that is strongly influenced by a whole range of lifestyle factors. Cholesterol is one of these factors, of course, but the modest effect of statins on mortality rates, even in large doses, reminds us that the current pharmacological approach has its limits and that we must definitely target other factors in the atherosclerosis process.

People who live in the Mediterranean basin have a risk of cardiovascular mortality on average much lower than those who live in northern Europe, even if their cholesterol levels are equivalent, just as an increase in cholesterol has only very little impact on the mortality risk of a Japanese person, whereas it causes a North American's risk to increase sharply (Figure 54). International variations in the incidence of cardiovascular disease are therefore not only due to cholesterol, but also reflect the importance of each culture's typical way of life.

In the same vein, a study of 136,905 patients admitted to hospital for coronary disease reported that up to 20% of them had optimal cholesterol levels, lower than 1.8 mmol/L. This illustrates how simplistic

HEART DISEASE MORTALITY IN VARIOUS PARTS OF THE WORLD

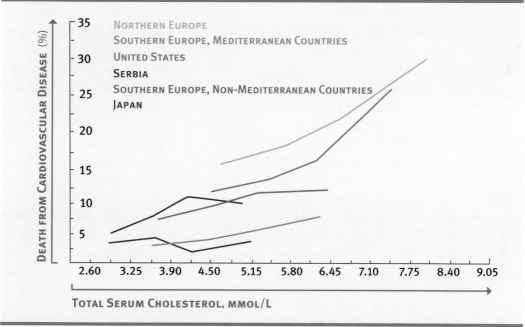

FIGURE 54

Source: Verschuren et al., 1995

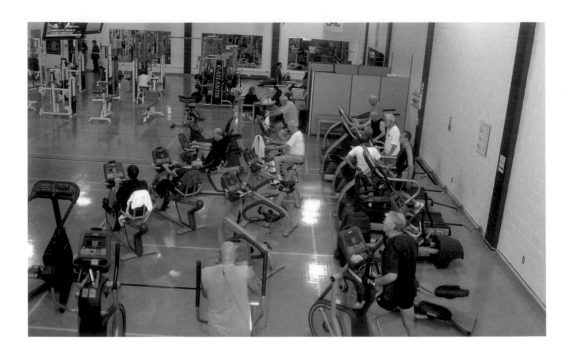

it is to aim mainly at cholesterol reduction to prevent coronary diseases.

Many of my colleagues tell me: "Changing habits is all very well, but, in real life, *no one* really wants to change their diet or get regular physical activity." I think nothing could be further from the truth. I'm far from convinced that people who are advised to take a statin for primary prevention and who are aware of the data on absolute risk reduction would be tempted to take a pill every day for the rest of their lives, knowing that they have about one chance in one hundred to benefit from it. When people are fully up to date on the scientific data and the remarkable benefits that diet and physical activity can have, and when they learn that these lifestyle modifications are much more effective than medication, most of them are prepared to make major changes in their lifestyle habits. I see this every day in my practice at the MHI's EPIC Centre.

Furthermore, medication can result in a false sense of security that discourages people from adopting better lifestyle habits. Every week, I hear patients say, "Since I've been taking a statin, I don't have to worry anymore about my diet, because my LDL cholesterol level is now 1.6 or 1.8." This way of thinking has serious consequences, as it gives the impression that a drug can counteract the effects of junk food on cardiovascular disease, obesity, diabetes, or cancer, which is false. This attitude is not just anecdotal. It has been well documented by two recent studies showing that statin users consume more calories, have a higher body mass index than those who do not take this class of drug and get less physical activity, probably owing to the negative impact of statins on muscles. This is very unfortunate, since reducing your cholesterol level with just a statin does not have the positive effects of a diet high in polyphenols, antioxidants, fibre, and anti-inflammatory substances (Chapter 4). Exercise also has many more benefits for overall health than do statins (Chapter 6).

A Typical Case of Statin Intolerance

I regularly see patients with quite severe side effects caused by statins. Recently, a patient consulted me about an arrhythmia problem, although he did not have any coronary disease, nor any risk factors for this disease. During our discussion, he explained that he had had to stop exercising 10 years before owing to muscle pains in his legs when he was walking. In addition, he had severe stiffness in the neck that greatly interfered with his driving: he felt pain when he turned his head to the side, which prevented him from properly checking the blind spot on his left. Gardening using his arms was also very painful.

After many medical visits and numerous physiotherapy sessions, he did not see any improvement. He attributed a weight gain of several kilograms to his sedentariness, since he had formerly walked 6 kilometres per day. As I had noted he was taking a statin (rosuvastatin, 10 milligrams a day), I asked him how long he had been using this drug and whether he had discussed the possibility of side effects with his doctor. The doctor had prescribed the statin 10 years previously and absolutely insisted the treatment continue, alleging that the discomfort was too "diffuse" and "non-specific."

I advised the patient to stop taking the statin for a week and call me back. This he did, telling me that his life had completely changed: the pains he felt when walking and after vigorous use of his arms had disappeared, as had the stiffness in his neck. As a result, he had begun walking 6 kilometres a day again and had resumed his gardening, among other activities. I advised him not to start taking this medication again, to continue his physical activities, and to choose a Mediterranean diet, which was not a problem for him at all. After six months, the patient had lost 6 kilograms and his waist circumference had decreased by 4 centimetres: his quality of life is completely different from before. And I'm convinced that he is at less risk now that he is eating better and getting more exercise than if he had continued his statin treatment. Although he's very happy, he's still extremely frustrated at having lost ten years of good quality life!

We must not lose sight of the fact that the main goal of various treatments (with statins or by other means) is not to attain a lower laboratory value (cholesterol level) but rather to prevent deaths, cardiac events, and strokes. We have to treat the patient, not a lab result. Based on my experience in secondary prevention and cardiac rehabilitation at the EPIC Centre, and after having seen thousands of patients, I can confirm that those who have modified their lifestyle usually have very favourable outcomes, even ten, twenty, or thirty years after their cardiac event.

As mentioned several times in this book, changing lifestyle habits can decrease cardiovascular disease risk by 80%. This is a protection that no drug will ever be able to provide.

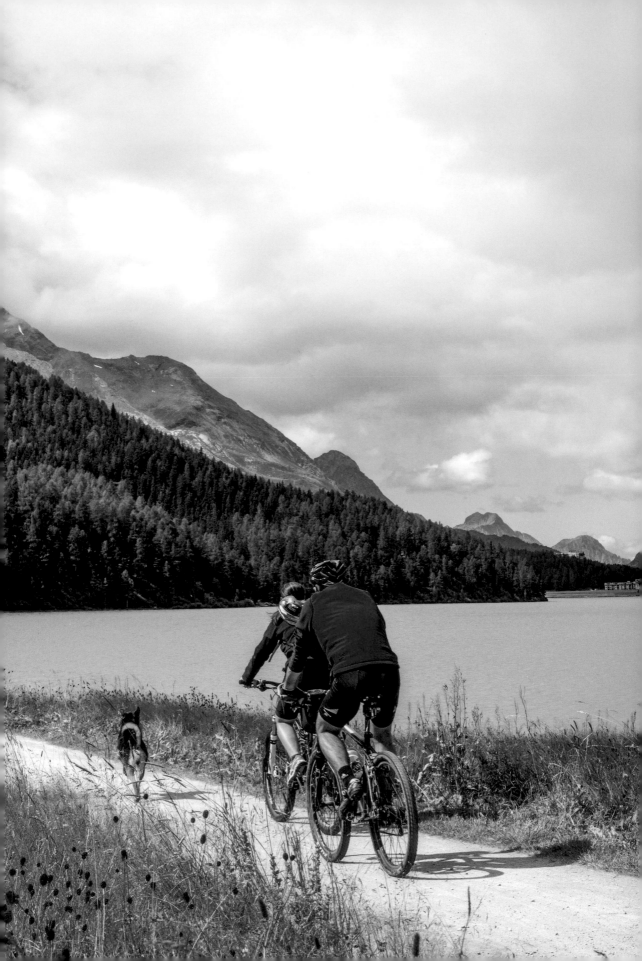

CONCLUSION

Since the beginning of the 1970s, there has been a rapid decline in cardiovascular disease of almost 50% in Western societies. We might have hoped, thanks to medical advances and prevention campaigns, that this decline would continue. Unfortunately, since the middle of the 1980s, we have been witnessing an unprecedented epidemic of obesity in every age group, and especially in children, adolescents, and young adults, which is causing a major increase in diabetes and other metabolic disorders. Not only do the gains of the last fifty years risk being erased, we now expect a further increase in the incidence of cardiovascular disease. Recent data from the United States confirm this prediction.

The only effective way to tackle the primary causes of cardiovascular disease is to fundamentally change our lifestyle.

In the case of smoking, the only thing to do is to quit: no sophisticated medical treatment is as effective as this solution. Similarly, no medical advance can replace the countless benefits of physical activity and better diet.

Changing lifestyle habits is a difficult undertaking that does not depend solely on individual choices: it requires the collaboration of all sectors of society to create environments conducive to health.

To Learn More ...

Introduction

Association pour la santé publique du Québec. *Bâtir la santé durable au 21ᵉ siècle.* 1–8. Montreal: ASPQ, 2016.

Gupta, Aakriti, et al. "Trends in Acute Myocardial Infarction in Young Patients and Differences by Sex and Race, 2001 to 2010." *Journal of the American College of Cardiology* 64, no. 4 (2014): 337–45.

Lloyd-Jones, Donald M. "Slowing Progress in Cardiovascular Mortality Rates: You Reap What You Sow." *JAMA Cardiology* 1, no. 5 (2016): 599–600.

Murray, Christopher J.L., et al. "Global, Regional, and National Disability-Adjusted Life Years (DALYs) for 306 Diseases and Injuries and Healthy Life Expectancy (HALE) for 188 Countries, 1990–2013: Quantifying the Epidemiological Transition." *Lancet* 386, no. 10009 (2015): 2145–91.

Sidney, Stephen, et al. "Recent Trends in Cardiovascular Mortality in the United States and Public Health Goals." *JAMA Cardiology* 1, no. 5 (2016): 594–99.

Chapter 1: Healthy Life Expectancy and Chronic Diseases

Akesson, A., S.C. Larsson, A. Discacciati, and A. Wolk. "Low-Risk Diet and Lifestyle Habits in the Primary Prevention of Myocardial Infarction in Men: A Population-Based Prospective Cohort Study." *Journal of the American College of Cardiology* 64, no. 13 (2014): 1299–306.

Boisclair, David, Yann Décarie, François Laliberté-Auger, Pierre-Carl Michaud. "Réduction des maladies cardiovasculaires et dépenses de santé au Québec à l'horizon 2050." *CIRANO* (2016): 1–13.

"Directly Measured Physical Activity of Canadian Adults, 2007 to 2011." *Statistics Canada.* Last modified November 27, 2015. www.statcan.gc.ca/pub/82-625-x/2015001/article/14135-eng.htm.

Ford, Earl S., Manuela M. Bergmann, Janine Kröger, Anja Schienkiewitz, Cornelia Weikert, and Heiner Boeing. "Healthy Living Is the Best Revenge: Findings from the European Prospective Investigation into Cancer and Nutrition—Potsdam Study." *Archives of Internal Medicine* 169, no. 15 (2009): 1355–62.

"Fruit and Vegetable Consumption, 2011." *Statistics Canada.* Last modified February 11, 2013. www.statcan.gc.ca/pub/82-625-x/2012001/article/11661-eng.htm.

Gierman, Hinco. J., et al. "Whole-Genome Sequencing of the World's Oldest People." *PLOS ONE* 9, no. 11 (2014): e112430.

Khaw, Kay-Tee, Nicholas Wareham, Sheila Bingham, Ailsa Welch, Robert Luben, and Nicholas Day. "Combined Impact of Health Behaviours and Mortality in Men and Women: The EPIC-Norfolk Prospective Population Study." *PLOS Medicine* 5, no. 1 (2008): e12.

Kirkwood, Thomas B.L. "A Systematic Look at an Old Problem." *Nature* 451, no. 7179 (2008): 644–47.

Lagacé, Patrick. "Je veux mourir à 69 ans." *La Presse*, January 20, 2016: http://plus.lapresse.ca/screens/302ab513-41f6-4718-bd0e-1469f1c62a92%7C_0.html.

"Leading Causes of Death, by Sex (Both Sexes)." *Statistics Canada.* Last modified March 9, 2017. www.statcan.gc.ca/tables-tableaux/sum-som/l01/cst01/hlth36a-eng.htm.

Loprinzi, Paul D., Adam Branscum, June Hanks, and Ellen Smit. "Healthy Lifestyle Characteristics and Their Joint Association with Cardiovascular Disease Biomarkers in US Adults." *Mayo Clinic Proceedings* 91, no. 4 (2016): 432–42.

Ludwig, D.S. "Lifespan Weighed Down by Diet." *JAMA* 315, no. 21 (2016): 2269–70.

May, Anne M., et al. "The Impact of a Healthy Lifestyle on Disability-Adjusted Life Years: A Prospective Cohort Study." *BMC Medicine* 13 (2015): 39.

Milot, Jean. "La mortalité infantile au tournant du XXᵉ siècle au Canada français." *Paediatrics and Child Health* 15, no. 5 (2010): e6–e8.

Normile, D. "Public Health: A Sense of Crisis as China Confronts Ailments of Affluence." *Science* 328, no. 5977 (2010): 422–24.

Oeppen, Jim, and James W. Vaupel. "Broken Limits to Life Expectancy." *Science* 296, no. 5570 (2002): 1029–31.

Olshansky, S. Jay, et al. "A Potential Decline in Life Expectancy in the United States in the 21st Century." *New England Journal of Medicine* 352, no. 11 (2005): 1138–45.

Ornish, Dean, et al. "Effect of Comprehensive Lifestyle Changes on Telomerase Activity and Telomere Length in Men with Biopsy-Proven Low-Risk Prostate Cancer: 5-Year Follow-Up of a Descriptive Pilot Study." *Lancet Oncology* 14, no. 11 (2013): 1112–20.

Popkin, Barry M. "Will China's Nutrition Transition Overwhelm Its Health Care System and Slow Economic Growth?" *Health Affairs* 27, no. 4 (2008): 1064–76.

Vita, Anthony J., Richard B. Terry, Helen B. Hubert, and James F. Fries. "Aging, Health Risks, and Cumulative Disability." *New England Journal of Medicine* 338, no. 15 (1998): 1035–41.

World Health Organization. "New WHO Report: Deaths from Noncommunicable Diseases on the Rise, with Developing World Hit Hardest." News release, April 27, 2011. www.who.int/mediacentre/news/releases/2011/ncds_20110427/en/.

Chapter 2: Coronary Disease and Its Treatments

Colles, Philippe, Martin Juneau, Jean Grégoire, Lucie Larivée, Alessandro Desideri, and David Waters. "Effect of a Standardized Meal on the Threshold of Exercise-Induced Myocardial Ischemia in Patients with Stable Angina." *Journal of the American College of Cardiology* 21, no. 5 (1993): 1052–57.

Juneau, Martin, Michael Johnstone, Ellen Dempsey, and David D. Waters. "Exercise-Induced Myocardial Ischemia in a Cold Environment: Effect of Antianginal Medications." *Circulation* 79, no. 5 (1989): 1015–20.

Meyer, Philippe, et al. "Exposure to Extreme Cold Lowers the Ischemic Threshold in Coronary Artery Disease Patients." *Canadian Journal of Cardiology* 26, no. 2 (2010): e50–e53.

Chapter 3: At the Heart of the Problem: Atherosclerosis

Allam, Adel H., et al. "Atherosclerosis in Ancient Egyptian Mummies: The Horus Study." *JACC: Cardiovascular Imaging* 4, no. 4 (2011): 315–27.

Angelini, Annalisa, Gaetano Thiene, Carla Frescura, and Giorgio Baroldi. "Coronary Arterial Wall and Atherosclerosis in Youth (1–20 Years): A Histologic Study in a Northern Italian Population." *International Journal of Cardiology* 28, no. 3 (1990): 361–70.

Aravanis, C., A. Corcondilas, A.S. Dontas, D. Lekos, and A. Keys. "Coronary Heart Disease in Seven Countries. IX. The Greek islands of Crete and Corfu." *Circulation* 41, no. 4 (1970): 88–100.

Berenson, Gerald S., Sathanur R. Srinivasan, Weihang Bao, William P. Newman, Richard E. Tracy, Wendy A. Wattigney. "Association Between Multiple Cardiovascular Risk Factors and Atherosclerosis in Children and Young Adults." *New England Journal of Medicine* 338, no. 23 (1998): 1650–56.

Brown, Michael S., and Joseph L. Goldstein. "A Receptor-Mediated Pathway for Cholesterol Homeostasis." *Science* 232, no. 4746 (1986): 34–47.

Chow, Clara K., Sanjit Jolly, Purnima Rao-Melacini, Keith A.A. Fox, Sonia S. Anand, and Salim Yusuf. "Association of Diet, Exercise, and Smoking Modification with Risk of Early Cardiovascular Events After Acute Coronary Syndromes." *Circulation* 121, no. 6 (2010): 750–58.

Després, Jean-Pierre. "Obesity and Cardiovascular Disease: Weight Loss Is Not the Only Target." *Canadian Journal of Cardiology* 31, no. 2 (2015): 216–22.

Enos, William F., Robert H. Holmes, and James Beyer. "Coronary Disease Among United States Soldiers Killed in Action in Korea: Preliminary Report." *JAMA* 256, no. 20 (1986): 2859–62.

Gaudet, Daniel, et al. "Relationships of Abdominal Obesity and Hyperinsulinemia to Angiographically Assessed Coronary Artery Disease in Men with Known Mutations in the LDL Receptor Gene." *Circulation* 97, no. 9 (1998): 871–77.

Glagov, Seymour, Elliot Weisenberg, Christopher K. Zarins, Regina Stankunavicius, and George J. Kolettis. "Compensatory Enlargement of Human Atherosclerotic Coronary Arteries." *New England Journal of Medicine* 316, no. 22 (1987): 1371–75.

Grundy, Scott M., et al. "Diabetes and Cardiovascular Disease: A Statement for Healthcare Professionals from the American Heart Association." *Circulation* 100, no. 10 (1999): 1134–46.

Kearney, Patricia M., Megan Whelton, Kristi Reynolds, Paul Muntner, Paul K. Whelton, and Jiang He. "Global Burden of Hypertension: Analysis of Worldwide Data." *Lancet* 365, no. 9455 (2005): 217–23.

Lewington, Sarah, et al. "Age-Specific Relevance of Usual Blood Pressure to Vascular Mortality: A Meta-Analysis of Individual Data for One Million Adults in 61 Prospective Studies." *Lancet* 360, no. 9349 (2002): 1903–13.

Libby, Peter, Paul M. Ridker, and Göran K. Hansson. "Progress and Challenges in Translating the Biology of Atherosclerosis." *Nature* 473, no. 7347 (2011): 317–25.

Liu, Kiang, et al. "Can Antihypertensive Treatment Restore the Risk of Cardiovascular Disease to Ideal Levels? The Coronary Artery Risk Development in Young Adults (CARDIA) Study and the Multi-Ethnic Study of Atherosclerosis (MESA)." *Journal of the American Heart Association* 4, no. 9 (2015): 1–12.

Lonn, Eva M., et al. "Blood-Pressure Lowering in Intermediate-Risk Persons Without Cardiovascular Disease." *New England Journal of Medicine* 374, no. 21 (2016): 2009–20.

Marmot, M.G., and S.L. Syme. "Acculturation and Coronary Heart Disease in Japanese-Americans." *American Journal of Epidemiology* 104, no. 3 (1976): 225–47.

Marmot, M.G., S.L. Syme, and A. Kagan. "Epidemiologic Studies of Coronary Heart Disease and Stroke in Japanese Men Living in Japan, Hawaii and California: Prevalence of Coronary and Hypertensive Heart Disease and Associated Risk Factors." *American Journal of Epidemiology* 102, no. 6 (1975): 514–25.

Mathieu, Patrick, Philippe Pibarot, Jean-Pierre Després. "Metabolic Syndrome: The Danger Signal in Atherosclerosis." *Vascular Health and Risk Management* 2, no. 3 (2006): 285–302.

McGill, Henry C., Jr., C. Alex McMahan, Edward E. Herderick, Gray T. Malcom, Richard E. Tracy, and Jack P. Strong. "Origin of Atherosclerosis in Childhood and Adolescence." *American Journal of Clinical Nutrition* 72, no. 5 (2000): 1307–15.

McNamara, J.J., M.A. Molot, J.F. Stremple, and R.T. Cutting. "Coronary Artery Disease in Combat Casualties in Vietnam." *JAMA* 216, no. 7 (1971): 1185–87.

Mozaffarian, Dariush. "The Promise of Lifestyle for Cardiovascular Health: Time for Implementation." *Journal of the American College of Cardiology* 64, no. 13 (2014): 1307–09.

Napoli, Claudio, Christopher K. Glass, Joseph L. Witztum, Reena Deutsch, Francesco P. D'Armiento, and Wulf Palinski. "Influence of Maternal Hypercholesterolemia During Pregnancy on Progression of Early Atherosclerotic Lesions in Childhood: Fate of Early Lesions in Children (FELIC) Study." *Lancet* 354, no. 9186 (1999): 1234–41.

Napoli, Claudio, et al. "Fatty Streak Formation Occurs in Human Fetal Aortas and Is Greatly Enhanced by Maternal Hypercholesterolemia: Intimal Accumulation of Low Density Lipoprotein and Its Oxidation Precede Monocyte Recruitment into Early Atherosclerotic Lesions." *Journal of Clinical Investigation* 100, no. 11 (1997): 2680–90.

Stamler, Jeremiah, Deborah Wentworth, and James D. Neaton. "Is Relationship Between Serum Cholesterol and Risk of Premature Death from Coronary Heart Disease Continuous and Graded? Findings in 356,222 Primary Screenees of the Multiple Risk Factor Intervention Trial (MRFIT)." *JAMA* 256, no. 20 (1986): 2823–28.

Sternby, N.H., J.E. Fernandez-Britto, and P. Nordet. "Pathobiological Determinants of Atherosclerosis in Youth (PBDAY Study), 1986–96." *Bulletin of the World Health Organization* 77, no. 3 (1999): 250–57.

Strong, Jack P., et al. "Prevalence and Extent of Atherosclerosis in Adolescents and Young Adults: Implications for Prevention from the Pathobiological Determinants of Atherosclerosis in Youth Study." *JAMA* 281, no. 8 (1999): 727–35.

Thompson, Randall C., et al. "Atherosclerosis Across 4000 Years of Human History: The Horus Study of Four Ancient Populations." *Lancet* 381, no. 9873 (2013): 1211–22.

Wilson, Peter W.F., Robert D. Abbott, and William P. Castelli. "High Density Lipoprotein Cholesterol and Mortality: The Framingham Heart Study." *Arteriosclerosis, Thrombosis, and Vascular Biology* 8, no. 6 (1988): 737–41.

Wright, Jackson T., Jr., et al. "A Randomized Trial of Intensive Versus Standard Blood-Pressure Control." *New England Journal of Medicine* 373, no. 22 (2015): 2103–16.

Zipes, Douglas P., and Hein J.J. Wellens. "Sudden Cardiac Death." *Circulation* 98, no. 21 (1998): 2334–51.

Chapter 4: Diet and Cardiovascular Disease

Abete, Itziar, Dora Romaguera, Ana Rita Vieira, Adolfo Lopez de Munain, and Teresa Norat. "Association Between Total, Processed, Red and White Meat Consumption and All-Cause, CVD and IHD Mortality: A Meta-Analysis of Cohort Studies." *British Journal of Nutrition* 112, no. 5 (2014): 762–75.

Alissa, Eman M., and Gordan A. Ferns. "Dietary Fruits and Vegetables and Cardiovascular Diseases Risk." *Critical Reviews in Food Science and Nutrition* 57, no. 9 (2015): 1950–62.

Astrup, A. "Yogurt and Dairy Product Consumption to Prevent Cardiometabolic Diseases: Epidemiologic and Experimental Studies." *American Journal of Clinical Nutrition* 99, no. 5 (2014): 1235–42.

Aune, Dagfinn, et al. "Whole Grain Consumption and Risk of Cardiovascular Disease, Cancer, and All Cause and Cause Specific Mortality: Systematic Review and Dose-Response Meta-Analysis of Prospective Studies." *BMJ* 353 (2016): i2716.

Bernstein, A.M., Q. Sun, F.B. Hu, M.J. Stampfer, J.E. Manson, and W.C. Willett. "Major Dietary Protein Sources and Risk of Coronary Heart Disease in Women." *Circulation* 122, no. 9 (2010): 876–83.

Brown, I.J., et al. "Sugar-Sweetened Beverage, Sugar Intake of Individuals, and Their Blood Pressure: International Study of Macro/Micronutrients and Blood Pressure." *Hypertension* 57, no. 4 (2011): 695–701.

Chen, G.C., et al. "Whole-Grain Intake and Total, Cardiovascular, and Cancer Mortality: A Systematic Review and Meta-Analysis of Prospective Studies." *American Journal of Clinical Nutrition* 104, no. 1 (2016): 164–72.

Crowe, Francesca L., et al. "Fruit and Vegetable Intake and Mortality from Ischaemic Heart Disease: Results from the European Prospective Investigation into Cancer and Nutrition (EPIC) Heart Study." *European Heart Journal* 32, no. 10 (2011): 1235–43.

de Koning, L., V.S. Malik, M.D. Kellogg, E.B. Rimm, W.C. Willett, and F.B. Hu. "Sweetened Beverage Consumption, Incident Coronary Heart Disease, and Biomarkers of Risk in Men." *Circulation* 125, no. 14 (2012): 1735–41.

de Koning, L., V.S. Malik, E.B. Rimm, W.C. Willett, and F.B. Hu. "Sugar-Sweetened and Artificially Sweetened Beverage Consumption and Risk of Type 2 Diabetes in Men." *American Journal of Clinical Nutrition* 93, no. 6 (2011): 1321–27.

Dhingra, R., et al. "Soft Drink Consumption and Risk of Developing Cardiometabolic Risk Factors and the Metabolic Syndrome in Middle-Aged Adults in the Community." *Circulation* 116, no. 5 (2007): 480–88.

Dietary Guidelines Advisory Committee. *Scientific Report of the 2015 Dietary Guidelines Advisory Committee.* Washington, DC: Department of Agriculture and Department of Human Services, 2015.

Du, Huaidong, et al. "Fresh Fruit Consumption and Major Cardiovascular Disease in China." *New England Journal of Medicine* 374, no. 14 (2016): 1332–43.

"Eating to live." *Scientific American* 16, no. 4 (2006): 1–89.

Fortmann, Stephen P., Brittany U. Burda, Caitlin A. Senger, Jennifer S. Lin, and Evelyn P. Whitlock. "Vitamin and Mineral Supplements in the Primary Prevention of Cardiovascular Disease and Cancer: An Updated Systematic Evidence Review for the U.S. Preventive Services Task Force." *Annals of Internal Medicine* 159, no. 12 (2013): 824–34.

Fretts, A.M., et al. "Consumption of Meat Is Associated with Higher Fasting Glucose and Insulin Concentrations Regardless of Glucose and Insulin Genetic Risk Scores: A Meta-Analysis of 50,345 Caucasians." *American Journal of Clinical Nutrition* 102, no. 5 (2015): 1266–78.

Fung, T.T., V. Malik, K.M. Rexrode, J.E. Manson, W.C. Willett, and F.B. Hu. "Sweetened Beverage Consumption and Risk of Coronary Heart Disease in Women." *American Journal of Clinical Nutrition* 89, no. 4 (2009): 1037–42.

Howard, B.V., et al. "Low-Fat Dietary Pattern and Risk of Cardiovascular Disease: The Women's Health Initiative Randomized Controlled Dietary Modification Trial." *JAMA* 295, no. 6 (2006): 655–66.

Hu, Frank B. "Plant-Based Foods and Prevention of Cardiovascular Disease: An Overview." *American Journal of Clinical Nutrition* 78, no. 3 (2003): 544–51.

———. "A Prospective Study of Egg Consumption and Risk of Cardiovascular Disease in Men and Women." *JAMA* 281, no. 15 (1999): 1387–88.

Ivey, K.L., J.M. Hodgson, K.D. Croft, J.R. Lewis, and R.L. Prince. "Flavonoid Intake and All-Cause Mortality." *American Journal of Clinical Nutrition* 101, no. 5 (2015): 1012–20.

Jakobsen, M.U., et al. "Major Types of Dietary Fat and Risk of Coronary Heart Disease: A Pooled Analysis of 11 Cohort Studies." *American Journal of Clinical Nutrition* 89, no. 5 (2009): 1425–32.

Johnson, Rachel K., et al. "Dietary Sugars Intake and Cardiovascular Health: A Scientific Statement from the American Heart Association." *Circulation* 120, no. 11 (2009): 1011–20.

Joshipura, Kaumudi J., et al. "The Effect of Fruit and Vegetable Intake on Risk for Coronary Heart Disease." *Annals of Internal Medicine* 134, no. 12 (2001): 1106–14.

Kaluza, Joanna, Agneta Åkesson, and Alicja Wolk. "Processed and Unprocessed Red Meat Consumption and Risk of Heart Failure." *Circulation: Heart Failure* 7, no. 4 (2014): 552–57.

Kromhout, D., E.B. Bosschieter, C. de Lezenne Coulander. "The Inverse Relation Between Fish Consumption and 20-Year Mortality from Coronary Heart Disease." *New England Journal of Medicine* 312, no. 19 (1985): 1205–09.

Lajous, M., A. Bijon, G. Fagherazzi, E. Rossignol, M.-C. Boutron-Ruault, and F. Clavel-Chapelon. "Processed and Unprocessed Red Meat Consumption and Hypertension in Women." *American Journal of Clinical Nutrition* 100, no. 3 (2014): 948–52.

Lajous, M., et al. "Flavonoid Intake and Incident Hypertension in Women." *American Journal of Clinical Nutrition* 103, no. 4 (2016): 1091–98.

Larsson, S.C., A. Akesson, and A. Wolk. "Egg Consumption and Risk of Heart Failure, Myocardial Infarction, and Stroke: Results from 2 Prospective Cohorts." *American Journal of Clinical Nutrition* 102, no. 5 (2015): 1007–13.

Levine, M.E., et al. "Low Protein Intake Is Associated with a Major Reduction in IGF-1, Cancer, and Overall Mortality in the 65 and Younger but Not Older Population." *Cell Metabolism* 19, no. 3 (2014): 407–17.

Li, Y., et al. "Saturated Fats Compared with Unsaturated Fats and Sources of Carbohydrates in Relation to Risk of Coronary Heart Disease: A Prospective Cohort Study." *Journal of the American College of Cardiology* 66, no. 14 (2015): 1538–48.

Libby, Peter, and Göran K. Hansson. "Inflammation and Immunity in Diseases of the Arterial Tree: Players and Layers." *Circulation Research* 116, no. 2 (2015): 307–11.

Liu, Rui Hai. "Health Benefits of Fruit and Vegetables Are from Additive and Synergistic Combinations of Phytochemicals." *American Journal of Clinical Nutrition* 78, no. 3 (2003): 517–20.

Lock, Karen, Joceline Pomerleau, Louise Causer, Dan R. Altmann, and Martin McKee. "The Global Burden of Disease Attributable to Low Consumption of Fruit and Vegetables: Implications for the Global Strategy on Diet." *Bulletin of the World Health Organization* 83, no. 2 (2005): 100–108.

Malik, Vasanti S., Barry M. Popkin, George A. Bray, Jean-Pierre Després, and Frank B. Hu. "Sugar-Sweetened Beverages, Obesity, Type 2 Diabetes Mellitus, and Cardiovascular Disease Risk." *Circulation* 121, no. 11 (2010): 1356–64.

Martínez-González, M.A., et al. "A Provegetarian Food Pattern and Reduction in Total Mortality in the Prevención con Dieta Mediterránea (PREDIMED) Study." *American Journal of Clinical Nutrition* 100, no. 6 (2014): 320–28.

Martínez Steele, Euridice, Larissa Galastri Baraldi, Maria Laura da Costa Louzada, Jean-Claude Moubarac, Dariush Mozaffarian, and Carlos Augusto Monteiro. "Ultra-Processed Foods and Added Sugars in the US Diet: Evidence from a Nationally Representative Cross-Sectional Study." *BMJ Open* 6, no. 3 (2016): e009892.

Mente, A., L. de Koning, H.S. Shannon, and S.S. Anand. "A Systematic Review of the Evidence Supporting a Causal Link Between Dietary Factors and Coronary Heart Disease." *Archives of Internal Medicine* 169, no. 7 (2009): 659–11.

Micha, Renata, Georgios Michas, and Dariush Mozaffarian. "Unprocessed Red and Processed Meats and Risk of Coronary Artery Disease and Type 2 Diabetes – An Updated Review of the Evidence." *Current Atherosclerosis Reports* 14, no. 6 (2012): 515–24.

Micha, R., S.K. Wallace, and D. Mozaffarian. "Red and Processed Meat Consumption and Risk of Incident Coronary Heart Disease, Stroke, and Diabetes Mellitus: A Systematic Review and Meta-Analysis." *Circulation* 121, no. 21 (2010): 2271–83.

Miedema, M.D., et al. "Association of Fruit and Vegetable Consumption During Early Adulthood with the Prevalence of Coronary Artery Calcium After 20 Years of Follow-Up: The Coronary Artery Risk Development in Young Adults (CARDIA) Study." *Circulation* 132, no. 21 (2015): 1990–98.

Minaker, Leia, and David Hammond. "Low Frequency of Fruit and Vegetable Consumption Among Canadian Youth: Findings from the 2012/2013 Youth Smoking Survey." *Journal of School Health* 86, no. 2 (2016): 135–42.

Mitka, Mike. "New Dietary Guidelines Place Added Sugars in the Crosshairs." *JAMA* 315, no. 14 (2016): 1440–41.

Moubarac, Jean-Claude, et al. "Processed and Ultra-Processed Food Products: Consumption Trends in Canada from 1938 to 2011." *Canadian Journal of Dietetic Practice and Research* 75, no. 1 (2014): 15–21.

Mozaffarian, D., T. Hao, E.B. Rimm, W.C. Willett, and F.B. Hu. "Changes in Diet and Lifestyle and Long-Term Weight Gain in Women and Men." *New England Journal of Medicine* 364, no. 25 (2011): 2392–404.

Mozaffarian, D., R. Micha, and S. Wallace. "Effects on Coronary Heart Disease of Increasing Polyunsaturated Fat in Place of Saturated Fat: A Systematic Review and Meta-Analysis of Randomized Controlled Trials." *PLOS Medicine* 7, no. 3 (2010): e1000252.

Pan, A., et al. "Red Meat Consumption and Mortality." *Archives of Internal Medicine* 172, no. 7 (2012): 555–59.

Pereira, M.A., et al. "Dietary Fiber and Risk of Coronary Heart Disease: A Pooled Analysis of Cohort Studies." *Archives of Internal Medicine* 164, no. 4 (2004): 370–76.

Price, Catherine. "The Cereal Box Is Lying to You — and So Is Every Other Label: Why You Can't Trust That 'Nutrition' Information." *Salon*, April 23, 2016. www.salon.com/2016/04/23/the_cereal_box_is_lying_to_you_and_so_is_every_other_label_why_you_cant_trust_that_nutrition_information.

Ramsden, C.E., et al. "Re-Evaluation of the Traditional Diet-Heart Hypothesis: Analysis of Recovered Data from Minnesota Coronary Experiment (1968–73)." *BMJ* 353 (2016): i1246.

Rohrmann, Sabine et al. "Meat Consumption and

Mortality: Results from the European Prospective Investigation into Cancer and Nutrition." *BMC Medicine* 11, no. 63 (2013): 1–12.

Routaboul, Jean-Marc, Steven F. Fischer, and John Browse. "Trienoic Fatty Acids Are Required to Maintain Chloroplast Function at Low Temperatures." *Plant Physiology* 124, no. 4 (2000): 1697–705.

Santé et des Services sociaux. *Plan stratégique du ministère de la Santé et des Services sociaux du Québec — 2015–2020*. Montreal: Santé et des Services sociaux, 2015.

Sinha, R., A.J. Cross, B.I. Graubard, M.F. Leitzmann, and A. Schatzkin. "Meat Intake and Mortality: A Prospective Study of over Half a Million People." *Archives of Internal Medicine* 169, no. 6 (2009): 562–71.

Siri-Tarino, Patty W., et al. "Saturated Fats Versus Polyunsaturated Fats Versus Carbohydrates for Cardiovascular Disease Prevention and Treatment." *Annual Review of Nutrition* 35 (2015): 517–43.

Soedamah-Muthu, S.S., et al. "Milk and Dairy Consumption and Incidence of Cardiovascular Diseases and All-Cause Mortality: Dose-Response Meta-Analysis of Prospective Cohort Studies." *American Journal of Clinical Nutrition* 93, no. 1 (2010): 158–71.

Song, Mingyang et al. "Animal and Plant Protein Intake and All-Cause and Cause-Specific Mortality: Results from Two Prospective U.S. Cohort Studies." *JAMA Internal Medicine* 176, no. 10 (2016): 1453–63.

Spence, J.D., D.J.A. Jenkins, and J. Davignon. "Dietary Cholesterol and Egg Yolks: Not for Patients at Risk of Vascular Disease." *Canadian Journal of Cardiology* 26, no. 9 (2010): 336–39.

Suez, Jotham, et al. "Artificial Sweeteners Induce Glucose Intolerance by Altering the Gut Microbiota." *Nature* 514, no. 7521 (2014): 181–86.

Swithers, S.E. "Artificial Sweeteners Produce the Counterintuitive Effect of Inducing Metabolic Derangements." *TEM* 24, no. 9 (2013): 431–41.

Tang, W.H.W., et al. "Intestinal Microbial Metabolism of Phosphatidylcholine and Cardiovascular Risk." *New England Journal of Medicine* 368, no. 17 (2013): 1575–84.

Virtanen, Jyrki K., et al. "Associations of Egg and Cholesterol Intakes with Carotid Intima-Media Thickness and Risk of Incident Coronary Artery Disease According to Apolipoprotein E Phenotype in Men: The Kuopio Ischaemic Heart Disease Risk Factor Study." *American Journal of Clinical Nutrition* (2016): 1–7.

Wang, Dong D., et al. "Association of Specific Dietary Fats with Total and Cause-Specific Mortality." *JAMA Internal Medicine* 176, no. 8 (2016): 1134–45.

Wang, Qiao-Ping, et al. "Sucralose Promotes Food Intake Through NPY and a Neuronal Fasting Response." *Cell Metabolism* 24, no. 1 (2016): 75–90.

Wang, Z., et al. "Non-Lethal Inhibition of Gut Microbial Trimethylamine Production for the Treatment of Atherosclerosis." *Cell* 163, no. 7 (2015): 1585–95.

Willett, Walter. "Diet Wars." *Frontline*, PBS, January 9, 2004. www.pbs.org/wgbh/pages/frontline/shows/diet/interviews/willett.html.

Yakoob, M.Y., et al. "Circulating Biomarkers of Dairy Fat and Risk of Incident Diabetes Mellitus Among U.S. Men and Women in Two Large Prospective Cohorts." *Circulation* 133, no. 17 (2016): 1645–54.

Yang, Q., Z. Zhang, E.W. Gregg, W.D. Flanders, R. Merritt, and F.B. Hu. "Added Sugar Intake and Cardiovascular Diseases Mortality Among U.S. Adults." *JAMA Internal Medicine* 174, no. 4 (2014): 516–19.

Zhu, Weifei, et al. "Gut Microbial Metabolite TMAO Enhances Platelet Hyperreactivity and Thrombosis Risk." *Cell* 165, no. 1 (2016): 111–24.

Zong, G., A. Gao, F.B. Hu, and Q. Sun. "Whole Grain Intake and Mortality from All Causes, Cardiovascular Disease, and Cancer: Clinical Perspective." *Circulation* 133, no. 24 (2016): 2370–80.

Chapter 5: Diet: Effects on Human and Planetary Health

CIHEAM/FAO. *Mediterranean Food Consumption Patterns: Diet, Environment, Society, Economy, and Health*. A White Paper Priority 5 of Feeding Knowledge Programme, Expo Milan 2015.

Conason, Joe. "Bill Clinton Explains Why He Became a Vegan." *AARP*, August/September 2013. www.aarp.org/health/healthy-living/info-08-2013/bill-clinton-vegan.html.

De Lorgeril, M. "Mediterranean Diet and Cardiovascular Disease: Historical Perspective and

Latest Evidence." *Current Atherosclerosis Reports* 15, no. 12 (2013): 370–75.

De Lorgeril, M., P. Salen, J.L. Martin, I. Monjaud, J. Delaye, and N. Mamelle. "Mediterranean Diet, Traditional Risk Factors, and the Rate of Cardiovascular Complications After Myocardial Infarction: Final Report of the Lyon Diet Heart Study." *Circulation* 99, no. 6 (1999): 779–85.

Esselstyn, C.B., G. Gendy, J. Doyle, M. Golubic, and M.F. Roizen. "A Way to Reverse CAD?" *Journal of Family Practice* 63, no. 7 (2014): 356–64.

Estruch, R., et al. "Primary Prevention of Cardiovascular Disease with a Mediterranean Diet." *New England Journal of Medicine* 368, no. 14 (2013): 1279–90.

Gould, K.L., et al. "Changes in Myocardial Perfusion Abnormalities by Positron Emission Tomography After Long-Term, Intense Risk Factor Modification." *JAMA* 274, no. 11 (1995): 894–901.

Greenpeace. *Ecological Livestock.* Amsterdam: Greenpeace International, 2013.

Huang, T., B. Yang, J. Zheng, G. Li, M.L. Wahlqvist, and D. Li. "Cardiovascular Disease Mortality and Cancer Incidence in Vegetarians: A Meta-Analysis and Systematic Review." *Annals of Nutrition and Metabolism* 60, no. 4 (2012): 233–40.

Hubbard, J.D., S. Inkeles, and R.J. Barnard. "Nathan Pritikin's Heart." *New England Journal of Medicine* 313, no. 52 (1985).

IPCC. "Summary for Policymakers." In *Climate Change 2014: Mitigation of Climate Change.* Cambridge: Cambridge University Press, 2014.

Key, T.J., et al. "Mortality in Vegetarians and Non-Vegetarians: A Collaborative Analysis of 8,300 Deaths Among 76,000 Men and Women in Five Prospective Studies." *Public Health Nutrition* 1, no. 1 (1998): 33–41.

Key, T.J., et al. "Mortality in Vegetarians and Non-vegetarians: Detailed Findings from a Collaborative Analysis of 5 Prospective Studies." *American Journal of Clinical Nutrition* 70, no. 3 (1999): 516–24.

Keys, A. "Mediterranean Diet and Public Health: Personal Reflections." *American Journal of Clinical Nutrition* 61, no. 6 (1995): 1321–23.

Martinez-Lapiscina, E.H., et al. "Mediterranean Diet Improves Cognition: The PREDIMED-NA-VARRA Randomised Trial." *Journal of Neurology, Neurosurgery, and Psychiatry* 84, no. 12 (2013): 1318–25.

McMichael, A.J., J.W. Powles, C.D. Butler, and R. Uauy. "Food, Livestock Production, Energy, Climate Change, and Health." *Lancet* 370, no. 9594 (2007): 1253–63.

Orlich, M.J., et al. "Vegetarian Dietary Patterns and Mortality in Adventist Health Study 2." *JAMA Internal Medicine* 173, no. 13 (2013): 1230–38.

Ornish, D., et al. "Can Lifestyle Changes Reverse Coronary Heart Disease? The Lifestyle Heart Trial." *Lancet* 336, no. 8708 (1990): 129–33.

Ornish, D., et al. "Intensive Lifestyle Changes for Reversal of Coronary Heart Disease." *JAMA* 280, no. 23 (1998): 2001–07.

Popkin, B.M. "Reducing Meat Consumption Has Multiple Benefits for the World's Health." *JAMA Internal Medicine* 169, no. 6 (2009): 543–45.

Salas-Salvadó, J., et al. "Prevention of Diabetes with Mediterranean Diets: a Sub-Group Analysis of a Randomized Trial." *Annals of Internal Medicine* 160, no. 1 (2014): 1–10.

Springmann, Marco, H. Charles, J. Godfray, Mike Rayner, and Peter Scarborough. "Analysis and Valuation of the Health and Climate Change Cobenefits of Dietary Change." *PNAS* 113, no. 15 (2016): 4146–51.

Steinfeld, Henning, Pierre Gerber, Tom Wassenaar, Vincent Castel, Mauricio Rosales, and Cees de Haan. "Livestock's Role in Climate Change and Air Pollution." In *Livestock's Long Shadow: Environmental Issues and Options.* Rome: FAO, 2009. 78–123.

Tilman, D., and M. Clark. "Global Diets Link Environmental Sustainability and Human Health." *Nature* 515, no. 7528 (2014): 518–22.

Toledo, E., et al. "Mediterranean Diet and Invasive Breast Cancer Risk Among Women at High Cardiovascular Risk in the PREDIMED Trial." *JAMA Internal Medicine* 175, no. 11 (2015): 1752–59.

Vermeulen, S.J., B.M. Campbell, J.S.I. Ingram. "Climate Change and Food Systems." *Annual Review of Environment Resources* 37, no. 1 (2012): 195–222.

Chapter 6: Exercise: The Best Medicine

Aizer, A., J.M. Gaziano, N.R. Cook, J.E. Manson, J.E.

Buring, and C.M. Albert. "Relation of Vigorous Exercise to Risk of Atrial Fibrillation." *American Journal of Cardiology* 103, no. 11 (2009): 1572–77.

Andersen, K., et al. "Risk of Arrhythmias in 52,755 Long-Distance Cross-Country Skiers: A Cohort Study." *European Heart Journal* 34, no. 47 (2013): 3624–31.

Avis du comité scientifique de Kino-Québec. *Quantité d'activité physique requise pour en retirer des bénéfices pour la santé.* Quebec: Ministère de l'Éducation et de l'Enseignement supérieur, 1999. www.kino-quebec.qc.ca/publications/QteActivitePhysique.pdf.

Benito, Begoña, et al. "Cardiac Arrhythmogenic Remodeling in a Rat Model of Long-Term Intensive Exercise Training." *Circulation* 123, no. 1 (2011): 13–22.

Bérubé, Nicolas. "Qualité de l'air: quand Montréal est pire que Pékin." *La Presse*, May 25, 2016. www.lapresse.ca/environnement/pollution/201605/24/01-4984763-qualite-de-lair-quand-montreal-est-pire-que-pekin.php.

Blair, S.N., H.W. Kohl III, R.S. Paffenbarger, D.G. Clark, K.H. Cooper, and L.W. Gibbons. "Physical Fitness and All-Cause Mortality. A Prospective Study of Healthy Men and Women." *JAMA* 262, no. 17 (1989): 2395–401.

Booth, Frank W., Christian K. Roberts, and Matthew J. Laye. "Lack of Exercise Is a Major Cause of Chronic Diseases." *Comprehensive Physiology* 2, no. 2 (2012): 1143–211.

Bramble, D.M., and D.E. Lieberman. "Endurance Running and the Evolution of *Homo*." *Nature* 432, no. 7015 (2004): 345–52.

Brook, R.D., et al. "Particulate Matter Air Pollution and Cardiovascular Disease: An Update to the Scientific Statement from the American Heart Association." *Circulation* 121, no. 21 (2010): 2331–78.

Brunner, D., and G. Manelis. "Myocardial Infarction Among Members of Communal Settlements in Israel." *Lancet* 2 (1960): 1049–50.

Brunner, D., G. Manelis, M. Modan, and S. Levin. "Physical Activity at Work and the Incidence of Myocardial Infarction, Angina Pectoris and Death Due to Ischemic Heart Disease: An Epidemiological Study in Israeli Collective Settlements (Kibbutzim)." *Journal of Clinical Epidemiology* 27, no. 4 (1974): 217–33.

CRTC. *Communications Monitoring Report — July 2011.* Ottawa: CRTC, 2011. http://publications.gc.ca/collections/collection_2011/crtc/BC9-9-2011-eng.pdf.

Daigle, C.C., et al. "Ultrafine Particle Deposition in Humans During Rest and Exercise." *Inhalation Toxicology* 15, no. 6 (2008): 539–52.

Defina, L.F., et al. "The Association Between Midlife Cardiorespiratory Fitness Levels and Later-Life Dementia: A Cohort Study." *Annals of Internal Medicine* 158, no. 3 (2013): 162–68.

Dunstan, D.W., et al. "Television Viewing Time and Mortality: The Australian Diabetes, Obesity and Lifestyle Study (AusDiab)." *Circulation* 121, no 3 (2010): 384–91.

Faselis, C., et al. "Exercise Capacity and Atrial Fibrillation Risk in Veterans: A Cohort Study." *Mayo Clinic Proceedings* 91, no. 5 (2016): 558–66.

Fries, James F. "Measuring and Monitoring Success in Compressing Morbidity." *Annals of Internal Medicine* 139, no. 5 (2003): 455–59.

Gillen, J.B., B.J. Martin, M.J. MacInnis, L.E. Skelly, M.A. Tarnopolsky, and M.J. Gibala. "Twelve Weeks of Sprint Interval Training Improves Indices of Cardiometabolic Health Similar to Traditional Endurance Training Despite a Five-Fold Lower Exercise Volume and Time Commitment." *PLOS ONE* 11, no. 4 (2016): e0154075.

Grøntved, A., and F.B. Hu. "Television Viewing and Risk of Type 2 Diabetes, Cardiovascular Disease, and All-Cause Mortality." *JAMA* 305, no. 23 (2011): 2448–55.

Guasch, E., et al. "Atrial Fibrillation Promotion by Endurance Exercise." *JACC* 62, no. 1 (2013): 68–77.

Guiraud, T., et al. "Optimization of High Intensity Interval Exercise in Coronary Heart Disease." *European Journal of Applied Physiology* 108, no. 4 (2010): 733–40.

Hakim, A.A., et al. "Effects of Walking on Mortality Among Nonsmoking Retired Men." *New England Journal of Medicine* 338, no. 2 (1998): 94–99.

Hankinson, A.L., et al. "Maintaining a High Physical Activity Level over 20 Years and Weight Gain." *JAMA* 304, no. 23 (2010): 2603–08.

Harris, K.M., J.T. Henry, E. Rohman, T.S. Haas, and B.J. Maron. "Sudden Death During the Triathlon." *JAMA* 303, no. 13 (2010): 1255–57.

Kim, J.H., et al. "Cardiac Arrest During Long-Distance Running Races." *New England Journal of*

Medicine 366, no. 2 (2012): 130–40.

La Gerche, André. "The Potential Cardiotoxic Effects of Exercise." *Canadian Journal of Cardiology* 32, no. 4 (2016): 421–28.

La Gerche, André, et al. "Exercise-Induced Right Ventricular Dysfunction Is Associated with Ventricular Arrhythmias in Endurance Athletes." *European Heart Journal* 36, no. 30 (2015): 1998–2010.

Lee, D.-C., R.R. Pate, C.J. Lavie, X. Sui, T.S. Church, and S.N. Blair. "Leisure-Time Running Reduces All-Cause and Cardiovascular Mortality Risk." *Journal of the American College of Cardiology* 64, no. 5 (2014): 472–81.

Matthews, C.E., et al. "Amount of Time Spent in Sedentary Behaviors and Cause-Specific Mortality in U.S. Adults." *American Journal of Clinical Nutrition* 95, no. 2 (2012): 437–45.

Maron, B.J., and A. Pelliccia. "The Heart of Trained Athletes: Cardiac Remodeling and the Risks of Sports, Including Sudden Death." *Circulation* 114, no. 15 (2006): 1633–44.

McGuire, D.K., B.D. Levine, J.W. Williamson, and P.G. Snell. "A 30-Year Follow-Up of the Dallas Bed Rest and Training Study: I. Effect of Age on the Cardiovascular Response to Exercise." *Circulation* 104, no. 12 (2001): 1350–57.

Moore, S.C., et al. "Association of Leisure-Time Physical Activity with Risk of 26 Types of Cancer in 1.44 Million Adults." *JAMA Internal Medicine* 176, no. 6 (2016): 816–25.

Paffenbarger, R.S., S.N. Blair, I.M. Lee. "A History of Physical Activity, Cardiovascular Health and Longevity: The Scientific Contributions of Jeremy N. Morris, DSc, DPH, FRCP." *International Journal of Epidemiology* 30, no. 5 (2001): 1184–92.

Paffenbarger, R.S., and W.E. Hale. "Work Activity and Coronary Heart Mortality." *New England Journal of Medicine* 292, no. 11 (1975): 545–50.

Paffenbarger, R.S., R.T. Hyde, A.L. Wing, C.C. Hsieh. "Physical Activity, All-Cause Mortality, and Longevity of College Alumni." *New England Journal of Medicine* 314, no. 10 (1986): 605–13.

Paffenbarger, R.S., M.E. Laughlin, A.S. Gima, and R.A. Black. "Work Activity of Longshoremen as Related to Death from Coronary Heart Disease and Stroke." *New England Journal of Medicine* 282, no. 20 (1970): 1109–14.

Panis, Luc Int, et al. "Exposure to Particulate Matter in Traffic: A Comparison of Cyclists and Car Passengers." *Atmospheric Environment* 44, no. 19 (2010): 2263–70.

Rowe, G.C., A. Safdar, Z. Arany. "Running Forward: New Frontiers in Endurance Exercise Biology." *Circulation* 129, no. 7 (2014): 798–810.

Saltin, B., G. Blomqvist, J.H. Mitchell, R.L. Johnson, K. Wildenthal, and C.B. Chapman. "Response to Exercise After Bed Rest and After Training." *Circulation* 38, no. 5 (1968): VII1–78.

Tuomilehto, J., et al. "Prevention of Type 2 Diabetes Mellitus by Changes in Lifestyle Among Subjects with Impaired Glucose Tolerance." *New England Journal of Medicine* 344, no. 18 (2001): 1343–50.

Verheggen, R.J.H.M., M.F.H. Maessen, D.J. Green, A.R.M.M. Hermus, M.T.E. Hopman, and D.H.T. Thijssen. "A Systematic Review and Meta-Analysis on the Effects of Exercise Training Versus Hypocaloric Diet: Distinct Effects on Body Weight and Visceral Adipose Tissue." *Obesity Reviews* 17, no. 8 (2016): 664–90.

Wang, B.W.E., D.R. Ramey, J.D. Schettler, H.B. Hubert, and J.F. Fries. "Postponed Development of Disability in Elderly Runners: A 13-Year Longitudinal Study." *Archives of Internal Medicine* 162, no. 20 (2002): 2285–94.

Wen, C.P., et al. "Minimum Amount of Physical Activity for Reduced Mortality and Extended Life Expectancy: A Prospective Cohort Study." *Lancet* 378, no. 9798 (2011): 1244–53.

Wen, C.P., J.P.M. Wai, M.K. Tsai, and C.H. Chen. "Minimal Amount of Exercise to Prolong Life." *Journal of the American College of Cardiology* 64, no. 5 (2014): 482–84.

Westerterp, K.R., and J.R. Speakman. "Physical Activity Energy Expenditure Has Not Declined Since the 1980s and Matches Energy Expenditures of Wild Mammals." *International Journal of Obesity and Related Metabolic Disorders* 32, no. 8 (2008): 1256–63.

Zhang, Hui-Jie, et al. "Effects of Moderate and Vigorous Exercise on Nonalcoholic Fatty Liver Disease." *JAMA Internal Medicine* 176, no. 8 (2016): 1074–82.

Chapter 7: Stress and Heart Disease

Akashi, Y.J., H.M. Nef, A.R. Lyon. "Epidemiology and Pathophysiology of Takotsubo Syndrome." *Na-*

ture *Reviews Cardiology* 12, no. 7 (2015): 387–97.

Allan, R. "John Hunter: Early Association of Type A Behavior with Cardiac Mortality." *American Journal of Cardiology* 114, no. 1 (2014): 148–50.

Baumeister, R.F., E. Bratslavsky, C. Finkenauer, and K.D. Vohs. "Bad Is Stronger than Good." *Review of General Psychology* 5, no. 4 (2001): 323–70.

Bybee, K.A., Prasad A. "Stress-Related Cardiomyopathy Syndromes." *Circulation* 118, no. 4 (2008): 397–409.

Cannon, Walter B. "Voodoo Death." *American Anthropologist* 44 (1942): 169–81.

Engel, G.L. "Sudden and Rapid Death During Psychological Stress. Folklore or Folk Wisdom?" *Annals of Internal Medicine* 74, no. 5 (1971): 771–82.

Frasure-Smith, Nancy, and François Lespérance. "Depression and Cardiac Risk: Present Status and Future Directions." *Postgraduate Medical Journal* 86, no. 1014 (2010): 193–96.

Ghadri, Jelena R., et al. "Happy Heart Syndrome: Role of Positive Emotional Stress in Takotsubo Syndrome." *European Heart Journal* 37, no. 37 (2016): 2823–29.

Kario, Kazuomi, Bruce S. McEwen, and Thomas G. Pickering. "Disasters and the Heart: A Review of the Effects of Earthquake-Induced Stress on Cardiovascular Disease." *Hypertension Research* 26, no. 5 (2003): 355–67.

Kitamura, T., K. Kiyohara, and T. Iwami. "The Great East Japan Earthquake and Out-of-Hospital Cardiac Arrest." *New England Journal of Medicine* 369, no. 22 (2013): 2165–67.

Leor, J., W.K. Poole, and R.A. Kloner. "Sudden Cardiac Death Triggered by an Earthquake." *New England Journal of Medicine* 334, no. 7 (1996): 413–19.

Lespérance, F., N. Frasure-Smith, M. Juneau, and P. Theroux. "Depression and 1-Year Prognosis in Unstable Angina." *Archives of Internal Medicine* 160, no. 9 (2000): 1354–57.

Ludwig, D.S., and J. Kabat-Zinn. "Mindfulness in Medicine." *JAMA* 300, no. 11 (2008): 1350–52.

Rosengren, A., et al. "Association of Psychosocial Risk Factors with Risk of Acute Myocardial Infarction in 11,119 Cases and 13,648 Controls from 52 Countries (the INTERHEART Study): Case-Control Study." *Lancet* 364, no. 9438 (2004): 953–62.

Rozin, Paul, and Edward B. Royzman. "Negativity Bias, Negativity Dominance, and Contagion." *Personality and Social Psychology Review* 5, no. 4 (2001): 296–320.

Schneider, R.H., et al. "Stress Reduction in the Secondary Prevention of Cardiovascular Disease: Randomized, Controlled Trial of Transcendental Meditation and Health Education in Blacks." *Circulation: Cardiovascular Quality and Outcomes* 5, no. 6 (2012): 750–58.

Skerrett, Patrick J. "The Science Behind 'Broken Heart Syndrome.'" *Harvard Health Publishing*, February 14, 2012. www.health.harvard.edu/blog/the-science-behind-broken-heart-syndrome-201202144256.

Yusuf, S., et al. "Effect of Potentially Modifiable Risk Factors Associated with Myocardial Infarction in 52 Countries (the INTERHEART Study): Case-Control Study." *Lancet* 364, no. 9438 (2004): 937–52.

Chapter 8: Tobacco and Electronic Cigarettes

CDC, OSH, and Health OOSA. *How Tobacco Smoke Causes Disease: The Biology and Behavioral Basis for Smoking-Attributable Disease.* Atlanta: CDC, 2010.

Doll, R., R. Peto, J. Boreham, and I. Sutherland. "Mortality in Relation to Smoking: 50 Years' Observations on Male British Doctors." *BMJ* 328, no. 7455 (2004): 1519.

Fagerström, Karl. "Nicotine: Pharmacology, Toxicity and Therapeutic Use." *Journal of Smoking Cessation* 9, no. 2 (2014): 53–59.

Fowler, J.S., et al. "Inhibition of Monoamine Oxidase B in the Brains of Smokers." *Nature* 379, no. 6567 (1996): 733–36.

Hurt, R.D., et al. "Myocardial Infarction and Sudden Cardiac Death in Olmsted County, Minnesota, Before and After Smoke-Free Workplace Laws." *Archives of Internal Medicine* 172, no. 21 (2012): 1635–37.

Peto, R., G. Whitlock, and J. Prabhat. "Effects of Obesity and Smoking on U.S. Life Expectancy." *New England Journal of Medicine* 362, no. 9 (2010): 855–57.

Prescott, E., M. Hippe, P. Schnohr, H.O. Hein, and J. Vestbo. "Smoking and Risk of Myocardial Infarction in Women and Men: Longitudinal

Population Study." *BMJ* 316, no 7137 (1998): 1043–47.

Royal College of Physicians. *Nicotine Without Smoke: Tobacco Harm Reduction.*" London: RCP, 2016.

Thun, Michael J., et al. "Lung Cancer Occurrence in Never-Smokers: An Analysis of 13 Cohorts and 22 Cancer Registry Studies." *PLOS Medicine* 5, no. 9 (2008): e185.

Chapter 9: Statins in Primary and Secondary Prevention

ALLHAT Officers and Coordinators for the ALLHAT Collaborative Research Group. "Major Outcomes in Moderately Hypercholesterolemic, Hypertensive Patients Randomized to Pravastatin vs. Usual Care: The Antihypertensive and Lipid-Lowering Treatment to Prevent Heart Attack Trial (ALLHAT-LLT)." *JAMA* 288, no. 23 (2002): 2998–3007.

Belluz, J. "How Bad Reporting on Statins May Have Led Thousands to Quit Their Meds." *Vox*, June 29, 2016. www.vox.com/2016/6/29/12057696/bmj-study-statins-media-influence-health.

Brown, M.S., and J.L. Goldstein. "Heart Attacks: Gone with the Century?" *Science* 272, no. 5262 (1996): 629.

Cannon, C.P., et al. "Ezetimibe Added to Statin Therapy After Acute Coronary Syndromes." *New England Journal of Medicine* 372, no. 25 (2015): 2387–97.

Cannon, C.P., et al. "Intensive Versus Moderate Lipid Lowering with Statins After Acute Coronary Syndromes." *New England Journal of Medicine* 350, no. 15 (2004): 1495–504.

Dehghan, M., et al. "Relationship Between Healthy Diet and Risk of Cardiovascular Disease Among Patients on Drug Therapies for Secondary Prevention: A Prospective Cohort Study of 31,546 High-Risk Individuals from 40 Countries." *Circulation* 126, no. 23 (2012): 2705–12.

Downs, J.R., et al. "Primary Prevention of Acute Coronary Events with Lovastatin in Men and Women with Average Cholesterol Levels." *JAMA* 279, no. 20 (1998): 1615–22.

Endo, A., M. Kuroda, and Y. Tsujita. "ML-236A, ML-236B, and ML-236C, New Inhibitors of Cholesterogenesis Produced by Penicillium Citrinum." *Journal of Antibiotics* 29, no. 12 (1976): 1346–48.

Heart Protection Study Collaborative Group. "MRC/BHF Heart Protection Study of Cholesterol Lowering with Simvastatin in 20,536 High-Risk Individuals: A Randomised Placebo-Controlled Trial." *Lancet* 360, no. 9326 (2002): 7–22.

Husten, Larry. "CardioBrief: FDA Panel Rejects Broader Ezetimibe Indication." *Medpage Today*, December 15, 2015. www.medpagetoday.com/cardiology/cardiobrief/55256.

Kollewe, Julia. "World's 10 Bestselling Prescription Drugs Made $75bn Last Year." *Guardian*, March 27, 2014. www.theguardian.com/business/2014/mar/27/bestselling-prescription-drugs.

Long-Term Intervention with Pravastatin in Ischaemic Disease (LIPID) Study Group. "Prevention of Cardiovascular Events and Death with Pravastatin in Patients with Coronary Heart Disease and a Broad Range of Initial Cholesterol Levels." *New England Journal of Medicine* 339, no. 19 (1998): 1349–57.

Majeed, Azeem, Paul Aylin, Susan Williams, Alex Bottle, and Brian Jarman. "Prescribing of Lipid Regulating Drugs and Admissions for Myocardial Infarction in England." *BMJ* 329, no. 7467 (2004): 645.

Mandrola, John. "Pivoting to Prevention and Population Health Will Not Be an Easy Pill to Swallow." *Medscape*, April 3, 2016. www.medscape.com/viewarticle/861389.

Matthews, Anthony, et al. "Impact of Statin Related Media Coverage on Use of Statins: Interrupted Time Series Analysis with UK Primary Care Data." *BMJ* 353, no. i3283 (2016): 1–10.

Mikus, C.R., et al. "Simvastatin Impairs Exercise Training Adaptations." *Journal of the American College of Cardiology* 62, no. 8 (2013): 709–14.

Nilsson, S., S. Mölstad, C. Karlberg, J.-E. Karlsson, and L.-G. Persson. "No Connection Between the Level of Exposition to Statins in the Population and the Incidence/Mortality of Acute Myocardial Infarction: An Ecological Study Based on Sweden's Municipalities." *Journal of Negative Results in BioMedicine* 10, no. 6 (2011): 1–8.

Ornish, D. "Statins and the Soul of Medicine." *American Journal of Cardiology* 89, no. 11 (2002): 1286–90.

Rea, Phillip A. "Statins: From Fungus to Pharma."

American Scientist (September–October 2008).

Sachdeva, A., et al. "Lipid Levels in Patients Hospitalized with Coronary Artery Disease: An Analysis of 136,905 Hospitalizations in Get with the Guidelines." *American Heart Journal* 157, no. 1 (2009): 111–17.

Sacks, F.M., et al. "The Effect of Pravastatin on Coronary Events After Myocardial Infarction in Patients with Average Cholesterol Levels: Cholesterol and Recurrent Events Trial Investigators." *New England Journal of Medicine* 335, no. 14 (1996): 1001–09.

Sampson, Uchechukwu K., Sergio Fazio, and MacRae F. Linton. "Residual Cardiovascular Risk Despite Optimal LDL-Cholesterol Reduction with Statins: The Evidence, Etiology, and Therapeutic Challenges." *Current Atherosclerosis Reports* 14, no. 1 (2012): 1–10.

Sever, P.S., et al. "Prevention of Coronary and Stroke Events with Atorvastatin in Hypertensive Patients Who Have Average or Lower-than-Average Cholesterol Concentrations, in the Anglo-Scandinavian Cardiac Outcomes Trial — Lipid Lowering Arm (ASCOT-LLA): A Multicentre Randomised Controlled Trial." *Lancet* 361, no. 9364 (2003): 1149–58.

Shepherd, J., et al. "Prevention of Coronary Heart Disease with Pravastatin in Men with Hypercholesterolemia: West of Scotland Coronary Prevention Study Group." *New England Journal of Medicine* 333, no. 20 (1995): 1301–07.

Sugiyama, T., Y. Tsugawa, C.-H. Tseng, Y. Kobayashi, and M.F. Shapiro. "Different Time Trends of Caloric and Fat Intake Between Statin Users and Nonusers Among U.S. Adults." *JAMA Internal Medicine* 174, no. 7 (2014): 1038–45.

Thompson, Richard, et al. "Concerns About the Latest NICE Draft Guidance on Statins." June 10, 2014. www.nice.org.uk/Media/Default/News/NICE-statin-letter.pdf.

Vancheri, F., L. Backlund, L.-E. Strender, B. Godman, and B. Wettermark. "Time Trends in Statin Utilisation and Coronary Mortality in Western European Countries." *BMJ Open* 6 no. 3 (2016): e010500.

Verschuren, W.M., et al. "Serum Total Cholesterol and Long-Term Coronary Heart Disease Mortality in Different Cultures: Twenty-Five-Year Follow-Up of the Seven Countries Study." *JAMA* 274, no. 2 (1995): 131–36.

Yusuf, S., et al. "Cholesterol Lowering in Intermediate-Risk Persons Without Cardiovascular Disease." *New England Journal of Medicine* 374 (2016): 2021–31.

Acknowledgements

I first want to thank Denis Gingras, who was an immense help to me in writing this book and without whom I would never have even tried to do so. His knowledge of basic science is an invaluable asset, along with his ability to summarize very complex concepts in simple terms.

I want to thank all the staff at the EPIC Centre and the Montreal Heart Institute, who do extraordinary work, and especially my secretary, Danielle Martel, whose able assistance ensured I had the undistracted time I needed to write this book.

My thanks go to Dr. Denis Roy, executive director of the MHI, who believed in the importance of this project and encouraged me to carry it out.

Thanks to Miléna Stojanac, of Éditions du Trécarré, who provided support for this work from the beginning.

Lastly, I would like to thank Dr. Judes Poirier, a great scientist for whom I have the utmost respect, for having convinced me to write this book.

About the Author

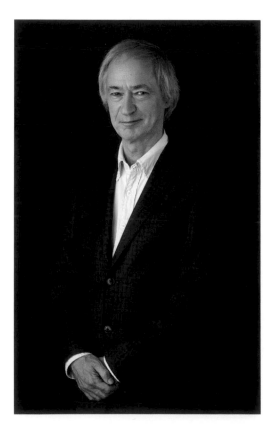

Director of prevention at the Montreal Heart Institute (MHI) and director and head of prevention and rehabilitation of the EPIC Centre, Dr. Martin Juneau lives in Longueuil, Quebec. Born in London to Canadian parents, he completed a Masters in clinical psychology at the University of Montreal in 1975 and subsequently did his medical studies at the Université de Sherbrooke. After a residency in cardiology in the University of Montreal network, he completed a fellowship in clinical research in the field of cardiovascular prevention at Stanford University in Palo Alto, California. On his return in 1986, he joined the Montreal Heart Institute as a clinical cardiologist and researcher, specializing in prevention and cardiac rehabilitation. He still practises general cardiology and preventive cardiology at the MHI, as well as at the EPIC Centre, which he has directed since 1988.

Dr. Juneau is also a clinical researcher who has published over 130 scientific articles and seven book chapters and given hundreds of lectures by invitation both in Quebec and internationally. A full clinical professor in the University of Montreal Faculty of Medicine, Dr. Juneau has held many positions, including that of chief of the Department of Medicine and Cardiology at the Montreal Heart Institute, director of professional services at the Montreal Heart Institute, and chair of the cardiology examining board for the Royal College of Physicians and Surgeons of Canada.

Dr. Juneau is a member of several boards of directors, including those of the Montreal Heart Institute Foundation and the Grand défi Pierre Lavoie. A founding member of the Canadian Association of Cardiac Rehabilitation, he has served as Quebec governor of the American College of Cardiology. He is also co-president, medical affairs, of Capsana, a company dedicated to prevention for the general public, affiliated with the Montreal Heart Institute.

He has been the recipient of many awards, including two from the Canadian Cardiovascular Society: the Robert Bamish Award in 2001, for the article that had the greatest impact on cardiology, as well as the Harold N. Segall Award in 2006, for his contribution to cardiovascular prevention in Canada. He received the Prix du mérite des Médecins francophones du Canada in 2011, the Prix du Professeur au mérite from the Department of Medicine in the Faculty of Medicine at the University of Montreal, also in 2011, and the Prix innovation sociale du Vice-rectorat à la recherche, à la création et à l'innovation at the University of Montreal in 2015.

His research interests are exercise and its applications in cardiology, sports cardiology, and the effect of cold and high temperature on patients with cardiovascular disease, as well as the role of stress in cardiovascular pathologies. Dr. Juneau preaches by example: a jogging enthusiast and passionate windsurfer, snowboarder, and downhill skier, he has followed a mainly vegetarian diet for over thirty years.

About the Epic Centre

The EPIC Centre is the centre for prevention and cardiac rehabilitation at the Montreal Heart Institute. Founded in 1974 by a group of patients who had participated in a study called the "Étude Pilote Institut de Cardiologie de Montréal" (Montreal Heart Institute pilot study) — hence the name EPIC — the centre was incorporated into the Montreal Heart Institute in 1983. Dr. Martin Juneau has been medical director since 1988.

The Montreal Heart Institute's EPIC Centre is the largest cardiovascular prevention centre in Canada, with over five thousand active members. Open to the public, it welcomes adults of all ages in primary prevention (with no cardiovascular pathology), as well as patients with cardiovascular disease (secondary prevention and cardiac rehabilitation).

The research team directed by Dr. Juneau at the EPIC Centre consists of cardiologists dedicated to prevention, exercise physiologists, kinesiologists, nurses, and nutritionists. The team also includes a large research group directed by neuropsychologist Louis Bherer, which is exploring the prevention of cognitive decline by improving lifestyle habits. The team of clinicians and researchers at the EPIC Centre have established the Montreal Heart Institute's Observatoire de la prevention (observatoireprevention.org, a website in French whose mission is to inform the public about major issues in cardiovascular prevention).

Photo Credits

François Escalmel: 28, 29, 30, 32, 34, 35, 37, 40, 43, 48, 51, 55, 61, 68, 75, 96, 116

Michel Rouleau: 122

Getty Images: Dean Mitchell/Getty Images 10; Sally Anscombe/Getty Images 12; Musketeer/Getty Images 14; Blend Images – KidStock/Getty Images 16; Marcy Maloy/Getty Images 19; Image Source/Getty Images 20; Image Source/Getty Images 21; Ascent Xmedia/Getty Images 24; Science Picture Co/Getty Images 25; Science Photo Library – ZEPHYR/Getty Images 26; Agence Photographique BSIP/Getty Images 29; Science Photo Library/Getty Images 31; jamesbenet/Getty Images 38; Associates – Biophoto/Getty Images 41; Vstock LLC/Getty Images 44; DigiPub/Getty Images 52; Martin Irwin/Getty Images 54; Rajko Simunovic/EyeEm/Getty Images 59; Janine Lamontagne/Getty Images 61; Yasuhiro Koyama/EyeEm/Getty Images 62; Gary S Chapman/Getty Images 69; Christine Birkett/EyeEm/Getty Images 73; John Block/Getty Images 74; Georgijevic/Getty Images 77; BRETT STEVENS/Getty Images 79; SHOSEI/Aflo/Getty Images 80; Jetta Productions/Getty Images 88; Bim/Getty Images 93; davidf/Getty Images 100; moodboard/Getty Images 98; Paul Bradbury/Getty Images 110; Dougal Waters/Getty Images 113; Alexandra Dudkina/EyeEm/Getty Images 118; Laurence Cartwright Photography/Getty Images 114; B. Boissonnet/Getty Images 122; Chris Gallagher/Getty Images 124; SolStock/Getty Images 131; James Leynse/Getty Images 133

Shutterstock: pixelaway 33; l i g h t p o e t 57; Anastasia Grankina 64; Joe Gough, 66; 5 66; Tatiana Popova, 66; amenic181 66; Mivr 81 valeriiaarnaud 60; Rawpixel.com 70; its_al_dente 83; Kuznetcov_Konstantin 86; Joseph Sohm 95; kart31 97; blurAZ 102; Rawpixel.com 104; Pressmaster 109; Iakov Filimonov 111; Dmitry Kalinovsky 112; Rommel Canlas 117; Image Point Fr 120; Kryvenok Anastasiia 135; Olaf Protze 140

Techniques Audiovisuelles ICM: 36, 84, 89, 136, 138

MixoWeb/EPIC Centre: 99

C.B. Esselstyn Jr.: 78

Harvard Health Publications: 108

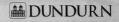
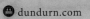